Not Dead Yet

Also by Julia Neuberger

The Moral State We're In

Not Dead Yet

A Manifesto for Old Age

Julia Neuberger

HarperCollins*Publishers*

HarperCollins*Publishers*
77–85 Fulham Palace Road,
Hammersmith, London W6 8JB

HarperCollins' website address is: www.harpercollins.co.uk

First published by HarperCollins*Publishers* 2008

1 3 5 7 9 10 8 6 4 2

© Julia Neuberger 2008

Cover author photograph © Derek Tamea

Julia Neuberger asserts the moral right to
be identified as the author of this work

A catalogue record of this book
is available from the British Library

ISBN-13 978-0-00-722646-7
ISBN-10 0-00-722646-2

Printed and bound in Great Britain by
Clays Ltd, St Ives plc

Mixed Sources
Product group from well-managed
forests and other controlled sources
www.fsc.org Cert no. SW-COC-1806
© 1996 Forest Stewardship Council
FSC

Contents

Dedication and acknowledgements

I could not have written this book without the extraordinary help and support of Ros Levenson, whose idea it was in part, who conducted much of the research, argued with me, briefed me, and generally helped me make it happen. Nor would it have been possible without the dedicated work of David Boyle, who took an unedited sprawling text and turned it into English – not to mention into manageable prose – as well as arguing through some of it at a late stage, and clarifying my ideas considerably. The team at HarperCollins has been supportive as ever – without Carole Tonkinson, Natalie Jerome, Jane Beaton and Belinda Budge, this volume would never have seen the light of day.

Huge thanks are due to my agent Clare Alexander, as well, dispenser of wise advice, firm encouragement, superb ideas, and lots of wine and sympathy, and to my assistant Paola Churchill, referred to by my whole family as 'my boss', because she tells me what I have to do, including finishing this book.

But this book would not have been possible without the help and support in quite other ways of my beloved parents, Walter and Liesel Schwab, wise to the end, whose old age I lived through with them and for them, of my uncle, Harry Schwab, and of my mother-in-law, Lilian Neuberger, who aged with astonishing grace and died at 94 whilst this book was in preparation. So *Not Dead Yet* is dedicated to their memory, as well as to my thoroughly alive and feisty aunt Anne Schwab, who is busy proving how effective you can be in old age – a lesson to us all.

When I was eighty-seven
they took me from my coffin;
they found a flannel nightshirt
for me to travel off in.

All innocent and toothless
I used to lie in bed,
still trailing clouds of glory
from the time when I was dead.

The cruel age of sixty-five
put paid to my enjoyment;
I had to wear a bowler hat
and go to my employment.

But at the age of sixty
I found I had a wife.
And that explains the children.
(I'd wondered all my life.)

I kept on growing younger
and randier and stronger
till at the age of twenty-one
I had a wife no longer.

With mini-skirted milkmaids
I frolicked in the clover;
the cuckoo kept on calling me
until my teens were over.

Then algebra and cricket
and sausages a-cooking,
and puffing at a cigarette
when teacher wasn't looking.

The trees are getting taller,
the streets are getting wider.
My mother is the world to me;
and soon I'll be inside her.

And now, it is so early,
there's nothing I can see.
Before the world, or after?
Wherever can I be?

'Run the Film Backwards', Sydney Carter

Introduction

Run the film backwards

It is a stabbing irony that as we become an elderly country we ignore the elderly with ever greater ferocity: if you don't look at the Ghost of Christmas Future, maybe it will never come.

Johann Hari, *Independent*, 19 January 2006

Dove contacted the manager of the sheltered accommodation where I live in Stoke Newington to see if there was anyone suitable. He told them about me and the casting director came round, but when I answered the door she pushed past and said, 'Is your mother here?' She didn't believe I could be 96 ... I was in Paris a fortnight ago, posing for a fashion magazine. Can you believe it?

Irene Sinclair, 97, the face of Dove soap

I am an only child, and I cared for both my parents as they got older and frailer. First, it was my father, though my mother did most of the caring, and talked constantly about how it was always the women who did the caring, and the women who were left behind. Later on, after my father's death, I cared for my mother, by then exhausted after looking after my father as he became sicker and more difficult. She had five more years as a widow, most of that time in extreme ill-health.

My experience – and that of countless friends and acquaintances – emphasizes both the best and the worst of caring for older people, and the way they are treated. It also makes it clear, if anyone had any doubts, that my mother was right. Benjamin Franklin first said: 'All would live long but none would be old', and he was right too. Or, as my mother put it: 'Don't get old – it's not much fun.'

There were good reasons why her final years were difficult. She was suffering from a rare chronic disease called Wegener's Disease, so rare that neither she nor I had ever heard of it before. As she became more infirm, she was very impatient about what she could no longer do. She became impatient with not being able to go back to work, feeling that her life now meant little. Certainly my mother was well cared for, and said so repeatedly. She even left us a letter saying so after she died. Yet she was miserable, felt superfluous, and could see no role for herself. This feeling seemed to be only partly linked to her health. She was very active and had large numbers of friends, but she still felt superfluous. Neither her friends, nor her grandchildren, nor her wider family were quite enough.

After she died, thinking over these things, I began to worry a great deal about the kind of society we have become, that allows older people to feel so miserable even when we try to provide all the care that they can need. It began to make me angry when I realized that she had been affected by the prevailing cultural view of people being old. She really felt, somehow, that she wasn't being noticed.

If that was the case, she didn't say so exactly. She kept saying that she had to go back to work. She had worked all her adult life, until she was 70. After that, she did a little bit of dealing in pictures, and was never somebody who did nothing. She seemed to feel, because she did not 'work' in the conventional way, that she had become a non-person. My experience since suggests that this feeling is very widely shared.

As the time passed after my mother died, the questions nagged away at me. I chaired an NHS trust that worked a great deal with older people, and – although the care was generally good – I found myself asking why older people's care had to be separate from other people's care. Of course older people tend to have multiple chronic issues, and there might be reasons why these should be treated together. Yet, in many parts of the UK, you get better care if you have a stroke when you are young than when you are old. There really is no excuse for that. It suggests that we think that lives are worth more when you are younger.

Also, why should my mother have felt so sidelined by society? Older people often used to feel they had an important role. They were the wise in society, the imparters of knowledge and experience to grandchildren. They provided stability in families that were troubled, and were often the carers of even older people, as well as being providers of comfort to those who were in pain or discomfort themselves. Other societies claim to maintain that role for older people. Some even manage it, some of the time, for some older people. But in modern Britain, those days seem to have gone completely. For my mother to argue that she wanted to return to work at the age of 82 means that she could not see what else there was for her without conventional paid work, in a culture that is increasingly obsessed with work.

Work gives purpose and meaning in our culture. We have failed to find the key to being less active, economically or purposefully, and still find meaning in life. 'What do you do?' is the question of choice, rather than 'Who are you and what are you like?' There was no clear way for my mother to be simply my mother – Liesel Schwab

– with all her expertise in art, her stories of life in Germany before the war, her accounts of being a refugee in London during the war, and her first few months in Birmingham before that. Her life, with its rich history and her hundreds of friends, was just not enough to satisfy her.

So my recent experience as a middle-aged carer of older people has convinced me we have got it wrong. More and more, it has made me feel we demean older people even when we do the best we possibly can under our present system. We make them feel worthless, past it, of no use, superfluous, as if they should have died years ago. When we give them help, we do things *for* them, rather than with them. More than anything else, this has made me question what it is to grow old in modern Britain and what it means to be an old person where old people are numerous and seen as a burden. It has also led me to ask whether we could make it any different.

I am certainly not the first person to formulate the questions in this way. Some of those conclusions have almost become truisms. Yet why are some of the basic changes that could be made, the most obvious ones – often relatively easy to achieve – still not being done? That, I believe, is what makes this book a little different. It recognizes that there are reasons, beyond the inadequacies of health policy or pensions policy, why we accept the inhuman situation for what it is, that we accept treatment for our older relatives that would cause an outcry if it was meted out to any other sections of society. It tries to stitch some of those reasons together and to come up with a practical way forward.

Because the real question is why we put up with this situation. If we look at our care system, still largely based on the Victorian Poor Law approach – assuming that the recipients should be grateful to get anything at all – we have to wonder why we don't get angrier about it than we do. We have to ask why we so rarely get furious about it, why we put up with it for parents and relatives and, unless we act quickly, for ourselves.

One of the experiences which opened my eyes almost more than anything else was the more recent decline of my uncle. He was Jewish, very orthodox, and gradually found himself unable to cope. It was never clear quite what was wrong with him, but he was becoming incontinent, and on the hospital ward kept on pulling his clothes off.

He would never have allowed anyone to see him naked, if he had been himself, and it was extremely distressing for us to see him acting in a way that was totally against every rule he had lived his life by. But when we raised this with the ward staff, they just said: 'Oh, we put clothes on him and he just takes them off again.'

They were not under-staffed. They could have asked about who this person they were treating was, and what he would feel about being allowed to wander around naked. If he kept taking his clothes off, then they ought to have discussed some practical solution, by sewing him in or clipping them on in such a way that they could not be taken off. They had objectified the people in their care, and had no sense of and no interest in who they were.

Of the four institutions which cared for my uncle before he died, one was different, and was the proof for me that something different is possible.

This was a London teaching hospital, about four miles away from the one which had performed so badly. It was very short-staffed, but my uncle was treated with incredible kindness before he finally began to slip away and became unconscious. Even then, the staff were going up to him and talking to him in case he could still hear. They didn't patronize him by calling him 'Harry'. It was clear to them that the person they were treating was a rather dignified old man, and they treated him as such.

But this story of inadequate, patronizing and inhumane care at the very end of life is reflected in the years before. What I want to do in this book is to look behind the immediate questions – why, for example, specific care is so poor – to ask something more fundamental. Is life as an older person in Britain today much fun? Are we thinking completely incorrectly about old people anyway by lumping them all together when, like everyone else, they could not be more different one from another? Does the state have a case to answer, or have old people themselves not been sufficiently voluble in the debates about pensions, care and costs?

This investigation is intended as a manifesto for old age. It asks whether, if we had 'run the film backwards' from old age to youth – as Sydney Carter suggests in his poem at the beginning of this book – we might see it all very differently. It also assumes that a generation will emerge, even if we are not quite there yet, which will simply not put up with what we have now. They – certainly we – will be impatient with excuses, demanding of services, demanding of other people, and, in short, as near an approximation to grey power as we are likely to see in the UK. We need to look inside ourselves and see why it is we accept such cruel and miserable lives for so many of our older people, our parents and – at the rate we are going – for ourselves. Many people lead wonderful lives as they get older. But when people don't, and when they end their lives in misery and degradation, it is we who allow it to happen.

The manifesto

This is the shape of the manifesto, and I will put some guts to it as each chapter goes by. Each chapter will end with a call to arms. What I want to see is an emerging 'grey power' movement, including all of us – old, young and middle-aged – who can make this happen. The chapters correspond to the key areas which need to be tackled:

1 Don't make assumptions about my age: end age discrimination

We need to have a clearer idea what constitutes a successful old age, and a sense of how that might differ from person to person. The mechanistic and medical definitions of professionals clearly don't sum up what might be very different experiences of various levels of physical ill-health and disability. Real people break out of those definitions but policy still traps them there.

That has to be set against new pictures of how we age and what we do at what stage of our lives. The age at which we have children is changing. Is 50 the new 30? Rates of teenage pregnancy in the past 20 years have never been higher in the modern era, but at the same time many women are delaying having their babies. The number of women having children in their thirties and forties has climbed steadily over the last 20 years, at a time when the overall birth rate has been dropping. In 2003, the fertility rates for women age 35–39 and over 40 both increased by almost 8 per cent.

As women may now be able to – and choose to – conceive well into their fifties and, eventually, perhaps beyond, older women may have sons and daughters who are going through the throes of adolescence or establishing themselves at work just at the time when the older person might need a bit of help, unless we are to live so much longer that dependent old age will not hit us until we are 95 or more. Indeed, from some 8,000 of us who reached 100 in 1997, there will be 30,000 or more in 2030 – and that is a relatively conservative estimate.

But it is easy to be blinded by the figures if we have no clear idea about what old age means, what we want from it, and how to get it, especially as we are likely to be treated – when the time comes – as if we have no opinions on the subject and are happy to sit in front of the television in our care homes.

2   Don't waste my skills and experience: the right to work

Then there are those issues about getting out into the world and playing an active role, which appears to be a basic human need at any age – and starting with the vexed question of appearances. Older people, and especially women, are always complaining about shops having no proper clothes for them, about how they hate communal changing areas – and swimming with younger, fitter people – and how they are always scared of being regarded as mutton dressed as lamb.

Any manifesto must insist on decent and accurate mirrors in shops, sales staff who are old enough to understand, single changing rooms, an alteration hand, and a decent range of clothes for the over-sixties. In exchange, older women would buy better clothes, check carefully that they were always well groomed – and therefore not 'invisible' as so many often complain – and keep up to date with emerging trends, as interpreted for older people.

The role models would be Joan Bakewell and Judi Dench and many, many more. But the fact that women are older – and men for that matter – does not mean they are not interested in their appearance, or that attractiveness and sexual attraction have disappeared. And headlines that suggest there was a plot to oust Menzies Campbell as Liberal Democrat leader for 'looking too old' are precisely those that depress, and anger, older people (he was a youthful 65 when that headline was published). It was particularly galling that the source who said this to the *Evening Standard* was quoted as adding: 'It's not that he is too old, it's just he looks too old ...'

That relates to getting out to work, but how many older people are going to continue to work into very old age? Should they have to? Is it only because pension provision and savings are so poor in the UK, or is there a better, or different, reason for older people working, to do with work giving meaning to life? And will that be full or part time? And will it be at the same status as previous jobs and careers, or at a lower status, however grand the title, as they often manage in the United States?

People want to be visible. Some older people want to work, some will need to because of the money, and many will need to be volunteers. What is essential is that older people are visible and welcome and being active. But that means adapting the rigid rules that now govern when they are allowed to do so, and bear little or no relationship to their actual abilities.

3 Don't take my pride away: end begging for entitlements

Then there is the question of money. The finer points of pensions are too abstruse and obscure for this kind of book, but what might older people expect as a basic minimum income, what might they be expected to pay for care out of that, and what things should be provided free or cheaper because people are older? Also, what is a reasonable proportion of wealth that should be left to our children?

Old age is not what it used to be. More of us will get there, and it is likely to last longer for most people than it used to. Better health and lower death rates mean that each successive generation is more likely to reach 65. Men now in their forties are nearly 90 per cent likely to collect their state pension, and the likelihood for women is over 90 per cent.

The concept of a long retirement is fairly new. The original state pension was set with a starting age where people were expected to live a few months or years, rather than several decades. This scenario of being retired for decades has many implications for financing old age, and that is where the political debate has tended to be. But it has equally important implications for people making choices about how they want to live, as well as around the support they may require. All over Europe, parents also want to pass their wealth onto their children and the children expect to inherit homes.

There are huge disparities and inequalities in income and wealth for older people. Some of this is sudden, brought about by old age and inadequate pension provision. In other circumstances, we see poor older people who have been poor all their lives, and then the question is whether we should try to redistribute older people's income to alleviate the worst of the misery in older old age.

Meanwhile, governments around the world, and particularly in Europe, are concerned at the effect the pensions 'time bomb' will have upon the wider society, and are using rhetoric that seems to blame older people for staying alive. Older people are becoming angrier about broken promises around financial and other support in old age, although arguably not angry enough, and younger people are beginning to fear what has hitherto always seemed to them to be impossibly far in the future.

4 Don't trap me at home because there are no loos or seats: reclaim the streets

Then there is the question of access to life, like the problem of transport and getting from place to place. Older people fill our buses and use their Freedom Passes with pleasure and abandon. What would an ideal transport system look like for older people when in rural areas many find it difficult to go anywhere if they do not drive, and in cities and towns there are still shortages of accessible transport, despite disability legislation? What would ideal transport look like? Would it be taxis, private car pooling, rental of wheelchairs in busy places, better access to buses, better and safer places to wait and sit at stations and bus stops?

Younger campaigners might find it awkward to talk about, but there is no doubt that the issue of public loos – as well as park benches, park attendants and seats in shops – are absolutely central to the way older people are being excluded from our town centres. Certainly, older people need to feel safe, given that many public spaces in cities feel as if they have been given over or abandoned to the young and disaffected. But unless there are adequate loos there as well, many older people feel they dare not leave their homes and go shopping. But because there seems an element of bathos about even mentioning it, nothing is done.

5 Don't make me brain dead, let me grow: open access to learning

What would it look like if education and educational activities were geared more to older people? Not only degrees, or the University of the Third Age, but specialist courses such as stone carving, pottery, art programmes and other things which could continue into very old – and possibly very frail – old age. Will university charges for degrees be reduced or waived for the very old, and should they be? Can older people get scholarships?

How can education work when some older people have problems with vision or hearing, and how well-adapted do universities and colleges, and general classes, have to be to help people hear and see all that is going on?

A fully inclusive educational programme might be geared less to future employment and more to the idea of education as fulfilment, as a goal in itself, to enrich one's life. So the instrumental view of education policy in many education authorities will need to be seen through a different, holistic lens that implies that education could and should be for its own sake.

6   Don't force me into a care home: real choice in housing

There is the basic question of accommodation, including people's own homes, sheltered housing, or – if things get rough – nursing homes and care homes, much feared by many older people and often rightly so. Nobody wants to give up their home and go into a 'home'. Yet questions about why we are still so bad at providing care at home, particularly – and maybe understandably – for older people with Alzheimer's disease, still need answering.

Fewer than one in twenty people want to spend their final days in a nursing home, yet one in five deaths takes place in those very places. We ought to be asking ourselves whether this is fair or right. Equally, there are questions around fitting homes for people who do become more frail and more disabled: why are architects and designers not putting real energy into designing for age? Why do older people seeking co-housing or mutual solutions find it so hard to make them happen, when they are commonplace in the USA and continental Europe?

7 Don't treat those who look after me like rubbish: train and reward care assistants properly

Then there is the question of care and support. Many older people need no more care and support as old people than they did when they were younger, but many do. Those with more money tend to buy that care in from private agencies. People with fewer resources are very dependent on local authorities, even though local authorities charge for the care they provide. What should be the quality of care provided in people's own homes or elsewhere?

How would we make it better, and how can we make sure there are no more stories about care workers coming to put people to bed at 6 p.m. or earlier? How can we teach local authorities that you cannot ask care workers to visit three or four older people in an hour, hour after hour, and carry out important personal tasks like toileting and putting people to bed?

What would care look like, if it were what people wanted, and what care workers often want to give, rather than what they get now? Indeed, what would it look like if those who look after old and frail people in their own homes, in sheltered housing or in care or nursing homes were treated quite differently? Care staff are poorly paid, poorly regarded, and have poor self-esteem. Perhaps the question that we should really ask is: what possesses us to leave our nearest and dearest in their care? And why are we not making a bigger fuss about the fact that care workers are badly paid and poorly regarded when often they do the most important, and often most difficult, of tasks?

8   Don't treat me like I'm not worth repairing: community beds and hospitals

There are certainly questions around health and healthcare, and how they operate for older people. How are decisions made, and who makes them? Who decides if older people are reasonably fit or not? How seriously are older people's own views about their state of health listened to? How far is it possible to get good generic care, without seeing too many specialists, as an older person? How easy is it to provide much of the care oneself? Who makes decisions about whether one should go for aggressive treatment or not? And how is it possible that hospital wards are so full of older people, of whom many seem to have no business to be there?

Would an ideal health system for older people look quite different, and have different rules? If so, would it be based on people's own advance directives and clear views about what they wanted themselves?

9   Don't treat my death as meaningless: the right to die well

We can hardly avoid the question about whether people can be allowed to reflect on meaning in life, and ultimately preparing for death. This is a curious section for the manifesto, but is essential: I have heard so much about how little space we allow for people to listen to older people making sense of their lives, telling their stories, recording life's meaning, one way or another. If you are perceived as useless, beyond your sell-by date, a 'wrinkly' with nothing to contribute, you will not be able to give voice to how your life has been, to make sense of it, to think it through, reflect on lessons learned, and plan for what you still want to do and what will be left undone, and how to come to terms with a certain amount of equanimity with one's impending death.

Some would call this space for spiritual awareness, and it is true that some people would find what they are looking for in this area in the churches and other faiths. But it goes further: we all need to make sense of our lives. We all need a sense of purpose, and indeed a sense of past and future.

Sydney Carter looked back at his life and ran though it, looking at himself at different ages and stages. For some of us, that is the way to do it. For others, it will be one particular aspect of life that will need emphasizing. Counsellors in hospices, and other staff in hospice and palliative care settings, often talk of how people try to put their affairs, and themselves, in order before they die. It cannot be beyond the wit of man and woman to invent or reinvent a space for this.

There are also questions about pain relief, and whether we recognize pain adequately – that pain is not always physical pain, but also spiritual, emotional and psychological pain. Dying people, most of whom are old, are enormously disadvantaged in our society, despite the relative popularity of hospices as a charitable cause. We have a tendency to shove dying people off to hospital rather than keeping them comfortable in their own space, and letting them die quietly at home. In the same way, why do we prefer invasive treatment – drips and forcible feeding – rather than gentle, hand-holding care?

10 Don't assume I'm not enjoying life, give me a chance: grey rage

Finally, part of this manifesto has to be the means to achieve all the rest, why we need to get angry and why we need a grey power movement to make it happen. Without this, discriminating against older people, and treating them less than well, will almost certainly continue. There is also a great deal to get angry about. People still have to sell their homes to pay for their care – opinions vary about whether that is reasonable – and people still get poor care when they have sold their homes, being moved time and again as nursing and care homes close. We still face violence against older people, far more than violence against children, but it barely makes the newspapers. Despite the brilliant stories of successful old age, we still allow so many older people to be ignored, degraded and driven prematurely into decrepitude and death.

There is no reason why older people should not be a very powerful generation. A long old age means that older people are significant consumers of a huge range of services, so their needs and tastes cannot be ignored. Politicians, one might have thought, need to heed the priorities of older people, not least because they turn out to vote more than younger people.

In fact, the pre-election period before the May 2005 election put older people on the political agenda for the first time. But they were neither sufficiently high on the agenda, nor taken seriously enough. It was also a disappointment to find that, despite the Conservatives' attempt to raise it, the pensions issue never really took off as central to the election campaign. Nor did long-term care, which has been a source of such resentment for many people; or even palliative care. All the parties said they would spend more, but no one said – as they should have done – that palliative care would be available for everyone who was dying, whatever condition was leading to their death.

But to start to use this latent consumer and political power we are going to have to deal with a whole range of hurdles. The media tend to go for stereotypes at the extreme – either the parachuting granny (isn't she amazing!) or the helpless and neglected old dear (what a tragedy!). For most of us, most of the time, we are neither parachuting, nor helpless – though some of us will have some time experiencing both phases. We need to find ways of breaking out of the traps that the stereotypes represent.

There is a range of obvious exceptions to start with. Older prisoners, older people who cannot get on with their families or neighbours, and older people who abuse vulnerable people, often their equally old partners, are not always the easiest to get along with, or even to provide services for. None of those fit the stereotypes. Nor do those older people who choose to live itinerant existences, travelling from place to place, staying only briefly, having no permanent roots and seeming to shy away from any kind of family or social involvement. Then there are those who move away for retirement, perhaps to a long-remembered, much-loved place associated with holidays as a child, despite the warnings of how difficult it is to make real friends as one gets older, and then proceed to lose touch with everyone they knew before, without making strong bonds in their new homes. Perhaps those are entrapping stereotypes too.

The stereotypes are the subtle ones that lead us to regard old age with fear and dread. Denial is a common response, both for people about to attain old age and for those who should be helping to plan services to meet their future needs. So time and again, when financial pressures hit health or social services, it is services for older people, community services, that get cut first. Less dramatic than closing acute wards, less vulnerable to bouts of shroud waving and cries of loss of life, the cuts of services to thousands of older people have a devastating effect. But because they do not feature in the planning, because of our habit of denial of getting old, being old and needing 'that little bit of help', those are always the first services to go. As the *Guardian* journalist Ray Jones put it so forcefully: 'A spiral of deteriorating performance is ... being created, with disabled and older people themselves being trapped in the vortex.'[1]

But that negativity seems to be shared by older people themselves. Research for the King's Fund suggested that people find it easier to discuss their wills than to discuss their care requirements with their families.[2] It is the same old fear and denial.

What is this about? Is it to do with our idea that human worth has something to do with economic productivity – and very narrow definitions of productivity too? We need to answer that question seriously as a society, and other questions too:

- Do we want to live in a society that does not take old people seriously, when so many older people are saying that at the end of their lives they become meaningless, and then they die?
- Do we think it acceptable to disregard people's wishes about where they want to die?
- Do we want to have, as an answer to extreme old age for some at least, euthanasia or assisted dying?
- Are we prepared to take on enough of the load of caring for extremely old and disabled people ourselves? Since we will never get any care system fully staffed, nor, probably, be prepared to pay for doing so even if the staff were available, this must be a young people's issue as well.

- Finally, are we ready to make a fuss about how people dying of anything other than cancer are treated?

We need to answer those questions because, if we can't, the misery will be greater, the anger will increase and we will be unable to do anything about it. That is why I have drafted this book in the form of a manifesto which answers those questions as I believe they must be answered. There will also be stories and care studies to illustrate the present position, plus some examples of what it might be like if things changed and we got the points in the manifesto recognized and acted upon.

I think this is a major political issue of the future, and a question of the kind of society we want to live in. Taken separately, many of the issues raised in the chapters that follow have been said before, but never quite angrily enough. We already have campaigns by the *Observer* and *Mirror* about dignity in old age. But they blame the healthcare system, which is simply looking at the symptom. The healthcare system is the way it is because we accept it – because many of us believe that, really, this abuse is OK.

The image of the old crone eking out her existence gathering sticks, bent double in freezing conditions, living in desperately poor housing, has largely disappeared from our consciousness – and so it should have. Yet perhaps it should not have disappeared completely, because we live with a modern version of that cruelty and neglect that may be different, but is just as shocking. The grey power campaign starts here and now.

Chapter 1

Don't make assumptions about my age

End age discrimination

Whatever you haven't done by your ninetieth birthday, you aren't going to do. Ever. Matron won't let you. And at almost every hundredth birthday the star of the show is a little old lady in a paper hat wondering why all these strangers are singing to her. I simply refuse to believe that nonagenarians enjoy watching the All New Scooby Doo Show *in the communal lounges every Monday afternoon. So let's see them on Saga outings bungee jumping until they reach the end of a long innings.*

Dr Mark Littlewood, *The Times*, **6 August 2005**

It had increasingly struck me that old people just get swept under the carpet and out of sight. Whether it's the half million living in care homes or the 3.5 million living alone. We really wanted to make old people visible again, and push them right back into the heart of society. What better way than to try and break them into the pop charts.

Tim Samuels, the documentary maker behind the rock band The Zimmers, BBC News, 28 May 2007

My father had heart disease for thirty years and, towards the end of his life, he found himself back in hospital at the point of death every 48 hours, suffering from chronic heart failure. As the sickness progressed, he kept finding himself at the distressing point where he could die at any moment. Eventually I had a conversation with his consultant, a lovely man called Dr Tom Evans at the Royal Free Hospital, who said: 'We could patch your father up again and he might get a bit longer, more like days or weeks rather than months, but I don't think it would be a kindness, because his suffering is getting much worse.'

He asked me whether he should tell my father this or whether I should. I chose to do so and it was a very difficult conversation. But I found that, although my father was very upset, he basically agreed. This was partly because of a sense that his generation shared that they had a finite claim on scarce health resources, but partly because each intervention was getting increasingly unpleasant. His inability to breathe was terrifying, and he was frightened of suffocating, and gradually becoming unable to do anything except feel increasingly angry at the situation he was in. The drugs were also having increasingly extreme side-effects. He itched all over, scratched himself raw, bled profusely and was desperately uncomfortable. He was also in a wheelchair going in and out of hospital. It was getting very distressing for him.

He was a feisty character and they could have kept him going longer, but we had a good doctor who decided – with my father – not to do so. My father could have disagreed, but in the end it wasn't an issue about the capabilities of medical science. It could have kept him alive a little longer, but for what?

That question – for what? – is at the heart of this chapter. This is not about euthanasia or killing people. It is to say that people need to have a sense of what kind of life they want, and just putting people back together for no purpose is not a kindness and, as I wrote in my last book – *The Moral State We're In* – we have become unkind in society because we have become so mechanistic. The question is increasingly 'Can we do it?' when it ought to be 'Should we do it?'

We *can* keep a lot of older people going for a long time with a very low quality of life. But the question of whether to do so should be discussed with them, so that when we treat them we do so with dignity and we understand their individuality and differences. If we don't do that, then professionals assume things on our behalf – either that we should be endlessly revived in the final days and weeks of our life, or that we could not possibly be enjoying ourselves and should not be treated at all. The danger then is that statistical assumptions will be made about our lives that decide officially and on our behalf whether our lives are worth living. There are many things that make life worth living, but we are increasingly allowing health economists – with their averages and statistics – to decide for us, and that is the root of a very serious unkindness indeed.

Longer lives

Retirement. Free time. A time to do what *I* want for a change. The end of the daily grind. No more nine-to-five or eight-to-four, and the exhaustingly long hours that we work in the UK compared to anywhere else in Europe. Most of us expect to get our pensions, whatever they are, however adequate or inadequate, when we are anything between 60 and 65. But our life expectancy has shot up dramatically, so that considerable numbers of us already make it to our century, and – if the government actuaries are to be believed – even more of us will do so in the not too distant future. But there is a peculiar contradiction in the way we think about the prospect of getting older. On the one hand, there is this escape from work responsibilities into a world of leisure; on the other hand, we are fearful of what lies beyond that – both individually and as a society.

Life expectancy in industrialized countries such as the UK has doubled over the past two centuries. More recently, life expectancy has also begun to rise across the developing world. In fact, most nations are experiencing continuous upward trends in longevity. But because of this contradiction, this astonishing feat – driven primarily by the successes of previous generations in combating early, preventable deaths – now evokes a curiously mixed response.

'It is hardly possible to open a newspaper without reading of the increase in life expectancy, and the consequently rapidly increasing proportion of older people in the population,' said the House of Lords select committee charged with reporting on the science of ageing.[1] 'More often than not these matters are considered for the economic impact they will have, be it on the cost of healthcare or on pensions. The underlying tone of such discussion is often negative, focusing on the 'burden' of increased numbers of older people and the threat of the demographic 'timebomb'.'

The 2001 Census showed that, for the first time, the number of people in England and Wales aged 60 and over was greater than the number aged under 16, but the figures for the 'oldest old' were even more striking. In 1951 there were 20,000 people aged 85 and over; by 2001 this had grown to over 1.1 million. Despite some considerable geographical and class variations, the trend is still upwards. Figures published in 2007 suggest that the life expectancy of women had shot up by 30 months in only four years to 85, while the gap between the top and bottom social classes had widened. Not quite an additional year of life expectancy for every year of life, but for those women in the professional classes a very different picture from the usual additional two years of life expectancy every ten years or so.[2]

Most observers and agencies concerned with forecasting future life expectancy used to predict that it would soon reach a plateau, when the gains from preventing early death had been consolidated. Then – or so they told us – the ageing process would settle down and we would see what it really was, stripped of early preventable deaths. But this never happened. Most evidence suggests that life expectancy within the UK and in other developed countries is still going up at the rate of about two years for each decade that goes by.

What is more, there is some evidence that it is speeding up. Studies in Sweden, where statistics have been kept since 1860, show that the increase in the age of the oldest person, far from slowing down towards a plateau, has been accelerating over the last 20 to 30 years. The UK government Actuary's Department predicted recently that there could be a million centenarians by 2074.[3] We are, in short, getting older and older.

Of course, these figures are based on the most optimistic life expectancy trends. If there is a serious flu pandemic, a late blossoming epidemic of BSE or a health decline due to obesity, it will not be quite so dramatic. Even the government actuary said the likely figure was nearer 350,000, which is still huge compared with the 10,000 or so centenarians now living in the UK. But people in their thirties now have a one in eight chance of living to be 100, and thousands could make it to 110, or even older.

There is still an academic disagreement about exactly what is going to happen. Emily Grundy, professor of demographic gerontology, has warned that the government has seriously overestimated, arguing that improvements in mortality rates in Denmark and the Netherlands have now stopped.[4] On the other side is the British Longevity Society's Myrios Kyriazis, who argues that the government is underestimating the numbers of us likely to reach 100. Like some American scientists, he believes that 'stem cell technology could completely transform how long future generations live by continually replacing our diseased organs, allowing us to surpass a thousand years.'[5] There are more bizarre predictions, especially among the futurist and IT community in the USA, which suggest we will soon be living to 5,000 years.

Similar arguments are going on around the world. There are already 25,000 centenarians in Japan, where there is a special 'Respect the Aged' day (19 September), when the latest group of centenarians is presented with a silver cup and a letter from the prime minister. Sri Lanka has an average life expectancy of 74.4 years, and Asian countries generally are shooting up the age expectancy tables, while Africa is showing a decline in age expectancy. Zimbabwe has a terrifying life expectancy of just 37.3 years and Botswana's is 35.5 years. These are results of a mixture of terrible governments, civil war, malaria and HIV/AIDS. But in most nations the trend is definitely upwards. The real question is going to be what this will mean.

If people live to 100 but still retire at 65, they will be retired – and presumably drawing a pension – for almost as long as they have been working. Some public sector occupations allow people to retire at 60 or even 55. I look more closely at the financial implications of getting older in a later chapter, and certainly pensions will affect how we live in retirement, but the real question is how we will judge success in our old age – and how policy-makers will define an old age well lived on our behalf.

There is a growing, though reluctant, consensus that we will have to work longer, which will postpone the age when old age officially begins. We will probably extend our working lives into our seventies or even eighties, though this may be done part time. But we will take those decisions partly based on the kind of older life we aspire to have – and the truth is that most of us seem likely to find ourselves there without having thought much about that. There is a paradox: as a society, we seem to be fearful of getting very old, yet at the same time want more and improved healthcare to keep us going longer. We fear retirement and worry about the financial resources, yet we resist working longer. We dare not, sometimes, even look too far into the future for fear of meeting ourselves there. It is a paradox that, in some ways, makes effective policy-making far more difficult.

'Ageism is worse than racism or sexism because there is so little recognition that it is wrong,' said Sohan Singh, 66:

> There is no commission fighting for your rights ... Ageing
> is a little bit like disability in that a lot of the problems
> are socially created. People may have more or slightly
> different needs as they get older, but the key thing is to
> keep people as human beings functioning as fully as
> possible. It is society that imposes on you a sense that you
> are old. I feel pretty young.[6]

In 2006, the journalist Stephen Moss interviewed eight centenarians in the *Guardian*, finding out about them in the pages of local newspapers.[7] He told their stories extraordinarily tenderly and respectfully. But there was a note of surprise in what he wrote, as if he never expected to find what he found. In his interviewing, he was left 'with one abiding impression: that they had been sustained by love – of parents, partners, and children. Most of all, partners, some long dead.'

It was, he said, 'much better than the usually quoted epigraph for extreme age – Shakespeare's "second childishness and mere oblivion, sans teeth, sans eyes, sans taste, sans everything".'

He did not find much in the way of regrets – 'the survivor's story was, at heart, a happy one' – though Moss felt that they did not always seem as happy as they said they had been. On the other hand, he wrote: 'They exhibited a stoic calm, an unshakeable acceptance of the hand that life had dealt them.'

They also lived for today. Harry Walker was asked what targets he still had in life, and replied:

> *There aren't any. You live day by day. I wake up in the morning and make sure that my legs are still working. I don't think I'm much trouble to the staff. I regularly go for a walk around the grounds. It's getting a bit harder, but I'm still living.*[8]

These centenarians, on the whole, despite some forgetfulness, some dementia, a stroke, various frailties and ailments, thought of themselves as relatively strong, healthy, and in good spirits – and one was still driving her car. Not a sad tale at all. It was a surprising story because society fears extreme old age, even fears the thought of so many very old people in our society.

We have two ways of looking at ourselves when old that are contradictory, said Mary Riddell in the *Observer* shortly after these interviews.[9] Are we 'British pensioners with double cataracts and leaking roofs', or are we the Greek goddesses to whom immortality is indispensable? Again, this contradiction seems to allow the treatment of older people in ways that we would never allow for someone younger. Mary Riddell cited the case of the British actors Francesca Annis and Ralph Fiennes. They had been together for eleven years; she was then 61, he a mere 43. The public was asked by the media to forgive Fiennes's affair with a singer on the grounds that Annis is 'so old' – and cheating on a long-term partner is clearly all right if she is old. Yet, if we are to live to 100 or more, 61 is barely middle age.

As for couples who are both elderly, they get treated with the greatest contempt. Like Richard and Beryl Driscoll, both 89 and married for 65 years, who were separated for seven months because Gloucestershire social services refused to pay for Mrs Driscoll to be in a care home alongside her frailer husband, even though she was blind.[10]

The question that Mary Riddell asked – What is all this extra life for? – is really the question at the heart of this book. Instead of allowing a gradual state of impermanence to take over – short-term marriages and relationships, constant cosmetic surgery, new ideas and yet more change – older people could call a halt to some of this, and ask the public at large to think again. But all this requires a real debate about what old age is for. Until we think about that a little more deeply, we will carry on treating older people as second-class citizens, and none of this will make much sense. And behind that question lies the issue of how we judge when old age is fulfilled and worthwhile, that state of being and aspiration which policy-makers call 'healthy life expectancy'.

Healthy life expectancy

But here there is a major problem. If life expectancy is rising, there is some evidence that healthy life expectancy – the years we spend well – is falling as a proportion. This is a vitally important discrepancy, if we believe it, because it would imply that more of our extra years will be spent sick and disabled in some way or other. That is the view of the Department of Health and the Office of National Statistics (ONS). But the ONS, at least, concedes that 'concerns remain about the reliability of subjective assessments ... They are known to vary systematically across population sub-groups ... [reflecting] differences in ill-health, behaviour, expectations and cultural norms for health.'

When the government responded to the 2005 report on ageing by a House of Lords select committee, they didn't mention these nuances. 'Although healthy life expectancy is increasing, it is doing so more slowly than overall life expectancy,' they wrote.

This irritated the select committee, which responded a year later by saying: 'this statement is made without any suggestion that it is either a cause of concern or that any remedial action is needed. It flies in the face of the claim by Professor Ian Philp, the National Director for Older People's Health, in a report published in November 2004, that "health in old age is improving and should continue to improve".'

So which is right? The National Director for Older People's Health? The Director of Research and Development for the Department of Health? The Office of National Statistics? How is the ordinary person supposed to make sense of this if three government departments face three different ways? Should we not be saying that we need to know, and that real research needs to be done, with longitudinal studies looking at people's health from the point of view both of experts and of older people, so that we know a little better what we are letting ourselves in for with all this increased life expectancy? Perhaps then we might make better decisions about it.

The ONS also gave an explanation, of sorts, for the apparent widening of the gap between life expectancy and healthy life expectancy. They say that people are getting more sensitive about their health, or have adopted higher expectations about their health, so that conditions that wouldn't have seemed like problems a few years ago are now considered to affect daily living. It may be that economic incentives are persuading people to think of themselves as ill more readily. There are theories, too, that improvements in survey methods have led to the discovery of a growing proportion of health problems.

Diseases are also being detected earlier, especially chronic diseases. People with ill-health are living longer. Illnesses and injuries that used to be resolved by dying are now more often managed instead. Short deadly illnesses, such as infectious diseases, have been replaced by diseases which are chronic and take a long time to resolve, if they ever do. Any of these could give the impression that healthy life expectancy was going down.

There is no doubt that feeling they are suffering from ill-health – even if they might be objectively no sicker than previous generations – would be quite enough to undermine people's quality of life and their sense of well-being. The question is what we can do about it. In their evidence to the House of Lords Committee, the Royal College of Physicians in Edinburgh warned that 'disability may be postponed but it cannot be eliminated'. That is obviously true. Nor can the adverse effects of disability be eliminated. But the question is whether it is possible to increase disability-free years in the UK, as they have in the United States, and how to reduce the adverse effects of disability on older people's lives?

At the moment it is hard to imagine how we can take on Professor Sir John Grimley Evans's advice to the House of Lords Committee on ageing. He said: 'Live longer, die faster'. That may be a wise piece of advice. But how do we put it into action, short of killing ourselves, something most of us don't want to do? And that's the stuff of another story, in another chapter.

If there is really an increase in ill health, nobody has ever explained it or measured it. The questionnaires that ask people to assess themselves on 'vague' concepts like health, while they may enable comparisons to be made with replies to the same questions from different groups or different areas, are not reliable enough to give us objective measures of health in old age. Perhaps the real question is whether the researchers are using sensible categories – and who, anyway, is deciding how people feel? Who is defining healthy old age?

Different definitions

This business of who decides if we are having a successful old age is important – and it is no small problem. One of the issues that has come up over and over again when I was researching this book has been the difference of approach between the 'experts' and the lay people, particularly those who are in fact old themselves, and have some experience to add to the picture. Behind that is the context in which these figures are generated.

We seem to have become caught in a technocratic idea in which the optimization of life expectancy together with the minimization of physical and mental deterioration is the only thing that healthy old age is all about. So the literature tends to focus on the absence of chronic conditions, on risk factors for disease, on levels of physical functioning – judged by others, rather than by older people themselves – and the extent to which their cognitive functioning is impaired. Alternatively, they may be quite healthy by objective standards and still beset by what Diana Athill describes as something more fundamental:

> *Our main trouble is that what he calls his 'weakness' – the*
> *dreadful draining away of energy from which he suffers –*
> *goes so deep that he has lost interest in almost*
> *everything.*[11]

Two British researchers, Ann Bowling and Paul Dieppe, reviewed all the literature for the *British Medical Journal*, and criticized this simple division between 'diseased' and 'normal', which they said was unrealistic.[12] There is a huge variety of conditions, of expectations of physical well-being, within all these groups. People see things differently and experience things differently.

To try to deal with this, two American researchers worked out a way of telling the difference between what they saw as usual ageing, with its normal decline in a variety of functions associated with age, and 'successful ageing' where people hang on to functions as much as they can.[13] They argued that there are three components of successful ageing:

- an absence or avoidance of disease and risk factors for disease
- keeping physical and cognitive functioning
- active engagement with life, including maintenance of autonomy and social support.

But that's not good enough either. There is a real problem with that definition as well. Most older people will not be disease-free. Many people begin their career of chronic, though not severe, disease in middle age. Trouble with hips and knees and sporting injuries leading to later arthritis are commonplace for people in their fifties and sixties, and earlier amongst keen sportspeople. Though they do not perceive this as the start of chronic disease, it often turns out to be just that – damaged joints lead to arthritis and other painful joint conditions. In just the same way, post-menopausal women often embark on a career of taking thyroxin for the rest of their lives, and other conditions of the skin or eyes, which tend to deteriorate quickly in late middle age, also begin to make their presence felt. So by the time people can reasonably be classified as older, in their late sixties or seventies – and with new projections of ageing perhaps even their eighties – there will be a great many so-called 'chronic conditions' at play. Add that the scares many women will have had with cancer – and some will actually have had and survived the disease – and you have a picture of older people who are certainly not 'disease-free'.

This description of being 'disease-free' is not a picture that means much to older people either, even if it means a great deal to medical experts who take a biomechanical model to assess ageing well. In one study, fewer than a fifth of older people can be demonstrated to be ageing well if these criteria are used.[14] Yet, if you ask them to assess themselves, around half of them say that they are, in fact, ageing very well, thank you.

Some have argued that it is easier to talk about disability-free life than about healthy life expectancy, and Sir John Grimley Evans was at pains to persuade the Lords select committee to take this different view, because 'it is disability and its associated loss of autonomy that older people fear, and which in turn leads to dependency with its cost implications for the health and social services'.

The trouble is that there are so many ways of estimating healthy life expectancy. It can be based either on self-assessed general health or self-assessed limiting long-standing illness. When it is a question of mortality, there is no doubt: deaths are formally registered. But when it comes to illness or disability, you have to get the information using a subjective assessment by the individual. And when it comes to information about rates of ill-health in the population, this is derived from the British General Household Survey, a nationally representative interview survey of residents in private households, conducted over many years. Each year about 25,000 individuals are interviewed, of whom around 4,000 are aged 65 and over. But the General Household Survey only includes people living in private households. Yet residents in communal establishments, care homes, nursing homes and sheltered housing and the like represent a significant proportion of the elderly and of those in ill health. The healthy life expectancy figures, on the other hand, are adjusted to take into account the health of residents in health and care institutions.

They also ask very different sort of questions. For the survey, people are asked questions like 'Do you have any long-standing illness, disability or infirmity?' For the Census, people are asked questions like 'Do you have any long-term illness, health problem or handicap which limits your daily activities or the work you can do (yes or no)'. For both the General Household Survey and the Census, people are asked: 'Over the last 12 months would you say your health has on the whole been good, fairly good or not good?'

We do get a little closer to what individuals actually feel with these questions, rather than what the definitions say they are supposed to feel – but not very much. There are concerns about this kind of subjective test, and whether one person's 'fairly good' is the same as someone else's, but there is a big plus: research shows that 'self-perceived health' is actually a good predictor of health outcomes. That being the case, there is good reason, despite the scientists' concern at the lack of objectivity, to trust the responses given by ordinary members of the public. They know how they feel and, apparently, their responses tie in neatly with their subsequent mortality, suggesting that the individuals concerned often had a clearer idea of what was going to kill them, and when, than the doctors did.

The difficulty comes in making comparisons with other countries, because they rely on different criteria. For example, the United States, Canada and Australia ask whether health is perceived as 'excellent, very good, good, fair or poor'. In those countries, those who perceive their health to be 'fair' are in the fourth category rather than the third. It is generally accepted that the prevalence of disability in later life has fallen in the United States since the 1980s, but we don't really know how this compares with this country. As far as the UK is concerned, 'the informed view is that we simply do not know what is happening, but there is certainly no evidence that disability levels in later life are falling as in the USA,' Sir John Grimley Evans told the Lords committee.

The benefits of using disability as a definition is that some international comparisons are possible. It is easier to define than ill health, but it is still far from being an absolute. Countries have different ways of defining what constitutes disability. Australia takes disability to be one or more of seventeen defined conditions. Japan takes disability to be confinement to bed. France includes as disabled all those in retirement homes. In the UK, disability is self-reported as a long-standing limitation on activities in any way.

So we still don't know, despite all the different ways of defining it, whether a healthy lifespan is increasing faster or more slowly than the lifespan itself. Yet the fact remains that, on any measure, there are a number of years – about eight in the case of men and eleven in the case of women – during which older people regard themselves as not being in general good health, or as having a limiting long-standing illness or disability. Such evidence as there is suggests that this period of perceived ill health is not decreasing, and may well even be increasing.

Life satisfaction and well-being

But it is even more complicated than that. Two other American gerontologists, Christopher Callahan and Colleen McHorney, took part in an academic retreat in Indianapolis to discuss successful ageing, and found an even wider difference in how 'experts' define success.[15] What emerged was that, for some scientists, health was the main – if not the only – definition of successful ageing. But for others it was something quite different and quite complex.

'To a humanist, health may be less relevant than realizing one's ambitions or helping a fellow human being to achieve his or her ambitions – neither necessarily requires health or longevity,' they wrote. 'If someone fulfilled the dreams of a nation, yet died of lung disease at aged 50 years, is that successful ageing?'

The narrow definitions of successful ageing may be inadequate, they said, but 'we may not have the tools to embrace the broader, more complex perspective'. The problem is that scientists, with their biomechanical, biomedical models, are not very good at complexity, and any discussion with older people – humanist or not – suggests that the scientific model is simply inadequate.

Callahan and McHorney say they want a new science of complexity, which they believe is just beginning to influence research on successful ageing. But their emphasis on humility is welcome. Because this is not only about complexity – though that certainly is a part of it. It is also about talking to older people and finding out from them what they think successful ageing is. Because, as sure as eggs is eggs, it is very different from the scientific, biomedical model.

One key element that Ann Bowling and Paul Dieppe cite in their article, based on a huge literature review, is that 'active engagement with life' is a key component in successful ageing.[16] 'Active engagement' is pretty difficult to define too, but there are some key elements to it. Top of the list are issues to do with autonomy and perceived autonomy. For many older people, the last thing they want to do, if they can possibly avoid it, is give up their home. It isn't that they necessarily love their own home, though many do; it is losing their autonomy that people so despair of, moving into a care home and not being allowed to take quite basic decisions for themselves.

If you have dementia, then there are relatively few alternatives if your family is unable to give you the care you need, particularly as the dementia advances. But with most kinds of physical frailty, people are determined to keep their autonomy, and will do a great deal to make sure they do so even if they do, sadly, have to go into residential or nursing care. That is why the best of the care and nursing homes do all they can to promote a sense of autonomy and give people a range of choices.

Along with the autonomy question – making decisions about when to go to bed and when to get up, when to eat, whether to go out or not, what programmes to watch or listen to – there are also questions about social engagement. The academic literature includes discussions about social, community and leisure activities, about social networks, support, participation and activity. But if you ask many older people what matters, as Stephen Moss's interviews made clear, it is love: love of a partner, even one maybe now dead, of children and grandchildren, siblings, friends and more distant family, an interest in the world. Often success means dealing with the world after the death of someone you love, as Katherine Whitehorn describes in her wonderful autobiography:

> *Being a widow is not helped by also being old. It's a relief, in a way, that my sagging curves no longer have an audience, but being on my own makes the prospect of being really ill and frail alarming. When I broke my wrist, there was Gavin to drive me to hospital and fasten my bra ... Losing your husband has two separate aspects: there's missing the actual man, your lover; his quirks, his kindness, his thinking. But marriage is also the water in which you swim, the land you live in: the habits, the assumptions you share about the future, about what's funny or deplorable, about the way the house is run, or should be; what Anthony Burgess called a whole civilization, a culture, 'a shared language of grunt and touch'. You don't 'get over' the man, though you do after a year or two get over the death; but you have to learn to live in another country, in which you're an unwilling refugee.*[17]

Bowling and Dieppe cite the theoretical definitions of successful ageing as life expectancy, life satisfaction and well-being (including happiness and contentment), mental and psychological health and cognitive function, personal growth, learning new things, physical health and functioning, independent functioning, psychological characteristics and resources, including perceived autonomy, control, independence, adaptability, coping, self-esteem, positive outlook, goals, sense of self, social community, leisure activities, integration and participation, social networks, support, participation and activity. But they point out that there are a whole range of extra lay definitions, including accomplishments, enjoyment of diet, financial security, neighbourhood, physical appearance, productivity and contribution to life, sense of humour, sense of purpose and spirituality – none of which are mentioned in the 'professional' literature at all. When you look at the categories that lay people added, they are the things that make anyone tick at any time of life: food and drink, sense of humour, a sense of purpose and, of course – much misunderstood by professionals – a sense of spirituality.

Even without those additions to the literature, much of the research shows that many of the areas of successful ageing are interrelated. Having a large number of social interactions and activities and lots of relationships is associated strongly with greater satisfaction with life and with generally better health and functioning better. Despite considerable class differences in survival and different attitudes according to the numbers of stressful events in life – such as loss of a partner or even a child – there are ways to make it easier for people to age well on their own terms, and according to their own values. Personal values, individual experience and a non-professional perspective are all key to defining what successful old age is for individuals. But a large part of that is about the nature of life, relationships, love and the ability to act.

So you have to give three cheers to Ann Bowling and Paul Dieppe's conclusion: 'Health professionals need to respect the values and attitudes of each elderly person who asks for help, rather than imposing our medical model on to their lives.'

The tyranny of a definition

Dr Muriel Gillick, a Professor of Ambulatory Care at Harvard Medical School, wrote one of the best reflections I have ever read on the subject of centenarians:[18]

Centenarians have something important to teach. Often they have wisdom arising from their accumulated experiences which they enjoy sharing, and which they are able to share because they aren't burdened by multiple maladies, each with its own demanding regimen of pills, monitoring tests, and physician visits. Their world is the antithesis of the elderly community in Florida, which has developed a culture that revolves around their health. The average elderly Floridian sees multiple specialists, often making more than one physician visit each week. Gathered around the table while eating an 'early bird special,' they exchange doctor stories. When one member of the group reports that he has seen a new specialist – perhaps a rheumatologist has joined the ranks of his cardiologist, urologist, and general internist – the others eagerly add the new doctor to their own list of 'providers.' In parts of Florida, the state with the largest elderly contingent in the United States, Medicare spends more than twice as much per capita for health care as it does anywhere else. What its citizens get in exchange for this largesse is more hospital days, more tests, more ICU admissions, and more subspecialty consultations in the last six months of life, with no evidence that the additional attention improves the quality of care.

But Professor Gillick says there is another lesson which is even more relevant to the question of definition:

The usual claim is that centenarians remain robust until a catastrophic event occurs, at which time, like the 'one-

hoss shay' of Oliver Wendell Holmes, they collapse
completely. Centenarians are different from other people
in that the ageing process has been postponed – at age
95, their organs are like those of a typical 75-year-old. But
there is no reason to believe that their organs are
programmed to fail simultaneously. The reason the
centenarian dies from his pneumonia or his heart attack
is that doctors do not aggressively treat their 100-plus-
year-old patients – they do not routinely admit them to
the intensive care unit, place them on a breathing
machine, start dialysis, or initiate any of the other
interventions that are commonplace in octogenarians.
Centenarians die quickly because we let them, and the
85-year-olds die slowly because we don't.

There are other ways in which our mechanistic definitions of old age undermine the health of older people. Far too many drugs are given to older people, quite inappropriately, wrote Dr Mark Copperfield, in his column in *The Times*, arguing that sensible older people refuse to take most of them, restricting themselves to 'the pink ones that stop their joints from aching'.[19]

But, he says, the trouble starts when they go into a care home, and matron insists on giving them the lot, promptly at 7 p.m., 'with predictable consequences'. Meanwhile, others who have been there longer are falling like ninepins, going to the hospital, having too many of all sorts of analgesics, sedating drugs, antidepressants and whatever.

Sir Richard Doll, who discovered the link between smoking and lung cancer, died at 92 and worked long past retirement, told pensioners not to expect NHS time and money to be spent on research into prolonging life, and advised them to 'live dangerously'. The alternative is that you will be defined according to a mechanistic definition of your age and treated accordingly.

Where we go wrong

So good health, and promoting independence, are key to any definition of being healthy for an older person him or herself. This sense of being in control, having the care we need and not being subject to other people's ideas of what would be just right for us, is critical for a sense of autonomy and well-being. You might have thought this fitted quite well with the ethos of the times, given all the mantras we hear about a patient-led NHS. Yet neither doctors nor patients are quite sure.

The patient-led NHS, with its huge emphasis on patient choice – which has to be a good thing in most circumstances – seems to have forgotten about continuity of care, about a personal relationship with the GP, about the small things that matter more than being able to choose where to have some particular procedure in middle age. Older people may need any number of procedures. What they don't usually need – or indeed want – is to have an isolated procedure done somewhere they have apparently 'chosen', apparently only on the basis of convenience or speed of access, but a long way from the care they get the rest of the time for their growing number of chronic conditions.

Diana Jelley, a GP in North Shields, puts this very well. There was a patient she had been looking after for some fourteen years, popping in to see her when she needed, a retired nurse who had had a heart attack aged 76 and whose condition gradually worsened over the years.[20] She was short of breath. She had heart failure. She had diabetes. She had high blood pressure. She had high cholesterol; her liver function was poor; and every intervention designed to improve one area of her disorders eventually ended up making another one worse.

'She is not the kind of patient who had the opportunity to fill in the "Your health, your care, your say" survey to inform the recent white paper on community care,' says Dr Jelley. 'But if she had been asked, I feel sure that continuity of care from a practice where everyone knew her was infinitely more important than the "instant access for routine care at any time" that seems to drive the White Paper'.

> But then she was not middle aged, middle class and living in middle England. She rated the quality of her personal care very highly – from the reception team to the visiting nurses and general practitioners. I don't think her view would have changed even if she had known that her care fell short in many areas of the Quality and Outcomes Framework indicators for which GPs receive payments as part of their contract. A few weeks ago she suffered another heart attack followed by a stroke, and never returned home. She died peacefully this week in a local 'continuing care' bed, at the age of 90. We had been on life's journey together over fourteen years – the epitome of what I had hoped and believed general practice would be about when I began my training at medical school.
>
> Last night, I opened her computer records to record a final entry: 'Goodbye to a true friend – RIP (Rest in Peace).' There are no longer any flashing alerts highlighting our failure to control her blood pressure, her ischaemic heart disease, or her diabetes. But then a smile overtook my tears. It was in true character that this generous spirited woman turned all the red entries green by dying just before the end of the financial year, when

figures count towards GPs' payment under this scheme.

I am not sure, as I approach retirement in another fourteen years' time, whether we will still be delivering this kind of care to our patients – quality that is very much appreciated but so hard to measure. Quality that means patients are looked after by 'my doctors and my practice'. Sections of the population quite understandably want a very different model of access and availability. But this focus may end up seriously eroding the delivery of long-term continuing care to the elderly and chronically sick. We are building our patient-led NHS. But sometimes I do wonder exactly which patients with which needs are actually *in the lead.*

It is not that older people just want to be able to choose everything for themselves, though they are no different from the rest of us in wanting control over their lives. It is that they want, when the time comes – when independence and choices are more difficult or impossible – to be able to have a relationship of trust with professionals who, ideally, they already know and to whom they have told those things that matter most to them when the going gets tough.

Call to arms

Who decides what old age ought to be like? Who measures it, and does it matter? The answer is that it almost certainly does matter, particularly given the wide disparity between 'professional' assessment and older people's own views. The gap between how professionals measure successful old age and how older people do it themselves is hugely important.

It suggests that older people have a more holistic sense of ageing well. But it also suggests – as is so often the case with professionals – that those factors which are harder to measure are somehow left off the list. Yet for all human beings, young and old, a sense of purpose in life is critical, however hard it would be to define and measure it. The question is: If we were to work out what it might mean to satisfy all of these criteria, those cited by professionals and by older people themselves, what might successful old age look like? That is what I want to explore in the chapters that follow.

It is an urgent task because there is such confusion out there. We all feel relatively certain that we want more years, but very uncertain what kind of years are possible. I don't want to die in my sixties, but I don't necessarily want to live through my eighties if my life is painful and meaningless. If it is all being done *to* me, or if I cannot process what is going on in my life, I might not feel that life is worth living. Especially if all I am able to do is watch game shows on TV.

As we get older, we begin to look towards the end of our lives, and make these calculations. Older people often say: 'I'm old.' They often say what they want to do, thinking about what time they have left and working backwards to see how possible it might be. They are constantly making calculations about what makes life worth living.

This isn't an issue about whether to end life. It is a question of how to measure its worth – to the person living it – so that they can take meaningful decisions. The point is that we need to help older people find ways of making life worth living and, when they get really ill – as my father did – allow them to discuss how much they want to keep being patched up.

But the tools policy-makers have for understanding these things, as we have seen, are very blunt. They use definitions which may be easy to measure but which are often completely irrelevant to individuals on the receiving end. Worse, they may use the tools of health economists – and their QALYS, or Quality Adjusted Life Years, the tools which purport to govern the rationing of healthcare – to decide about how to treat individuals.

QALYS and other forms of measurement can be extraordinarily useful when it comes to setting policy about where best to concentrate public money, but they are completely useless for individuals. Policy-makers need to stand back from community decisions when they are talking about individuals, but as managers take increasing control of these decisions the room for manoeuvre given to the poor health professionals gets ever smaller.

So that is what should go first into the manifesto: **Don't make assumptions about people's age, and what they believe makes life worth living – and therefore what resources they need and deserve – and end discrimination on the basis of age.** People are capable of doing and enjoying things until widely different ages. They are quite capable of working, and of making a unique contribution – even if it is just to those closest to them – for decades after the assumptions policy-makers make about them. This is a core message of this book. The manifesto also needs to include demands to:

- **Give guidance to health professionals to ignore QALYS and focus on the individual before them.** We have to give clinicians the chance to have a conversation with individuals and their families about their lives as they get older, to focus on what they feel is important, not what the policy says they should feel. The more we make our definitions of successful old age mechanistic, the harder it is for these conversations to take place.

Many older people do not want much more money spent on them. They simply want to be able to live as good a life as possible, and health professionals need to be able to discuss with them the best that they can do – individually.

Dumping QALYS as a tool for individual doctors means that they must take older people's *own* definition of their health status more seriously than the so-called objective status calculation of professionals. Unless they have dementia, older people know how they feel.

- **Force health and social care professionals to recognize the importance of love to older people, and make it deeply unethical to break or hamper people's relationships.** The separation of long-standing married couples when they were forced to go into workhouses was one of the main criticisms of the institutions in Victorian Britain. If we continue to divide married couples against their will because of shortcomings in budgets or institutions, then we have returned to that level of degradation. It is also extremely short-sighted. Nothing is more likely to hasten people's physical decline, and make them more dependent on scarce services, than dividing them from those they love.

- **Provide proper support for family carers.** The role of informal family carers has had far greater exposure in recent years as a result of the astonishingly successful campaigning by Carers UK and others. Carers and family members, often spouses and partners, but also children and siblings, give years of unpaid service. They save the exchequer billions every year. If health and social care professionals took the role of carers seriously, and understood how important love is in the functioning of older people, then carers would be better supported, respite care would be available to give everyone a break, and further paid support would be provided when the old person went home again.

Chapter 2

Don't waste my skills and experience

The right to work

It is now a generally accepted fact that old age stinks, and in some ways it does. I know because I've seen my mother go through it and now I'm getting there: my top lip is disappearing, my whiskers are growing, my hair is grey, my moles are mushrooming, I've lost what good looks I ever had, and when I had them I didn't really know it and now they're gone for ever, but would I give a toss if beauty wasn't so vital and wrinkled women were all over the papers?

Michele Hanson, *Guardian*, 30 August 2006

The internet is not just for people in their twenties ... I was pretty ancient when I got my first computer. Dear old ladies like me can take it up.

Jacquie Lawson, who became the market leader in online greeting cards at the age of 62

One of the things my mother used to say she hated most about getting old is that she didn't like the way she looked. My mother had been saying she had the worst legs in London right through her life. Now that she had the most terrible wasting disease, which made her lose a great deal of weight and made her legs extremely painful, she looked down at them, and said – with a twinkle in her eye – that they were finally 'improving'.

I tell this story because it illustrates a little of just how conscious older people are about their appearance. My mother's legs gave her a great deal of pain, but she was able to derive some rueful satisfaction from the fact that they were finally a little slimmer.

Nor is she alone in this. If you look at some of the books of advice about getting old, there is always a great deal there about appearance, and the importance of 'not letting yourself go'. This is advice aimed particularly at women, but it also applies to men, who find themselves all too easily in a combination of trainers and track suit bottoms, just because they are easier – for them or their carers – to put on and take off.

Older people feel that appearance is important, and they are right. Partly this is about self-respect, partly it is some protection against being treated like some dotty old biddy. This chapter is about work in the broadest sense. It is about being out in the world. That might seem a million miles from the question of appearance for younger people, but for older people the two are very much intertwined. Being active in the world, and *appearing* to be active in the world, are both prerequisites for self-respect, and for respect too in a society which is deeply biased against the old. That means underpinning your life by having a purpose and a reason for getting out of bed every morning, and looking as if you do too. Of all the aspects of life for older people in this book, these are the most important for them, and the most likely to keep people healthy for longer: looking as if you deserve respect, as well as having a role that brings respect.

In fact, of all the areas I talked to people about when I was researching this book, the issue of physical appearance probably provoked the most discussion amongst family and friends, not to mention the variety of experts. Actually, most of them agreed. On the one hand, most people felt it wasn't a good idea to let yourself go. On the other, there was a clear view about how important it was to keep your self-respect, which meant staying looking good, being attractive to other people.

It did not just mean something sexual. It was also important to look good to be attractive to nurse, visit or simply be someone to be wheeled out for the grandchildren. But it was an opinion that was widely shared among older people themselves. The fact that their own definition of ageing well involves looking good suggests that this is hugely important to some older people, if not all of them. Some undoubtedly feel that being older means you can give up on the diet, abuse the body and wear tracksuits day in and day out. But it is hard to escape the bombardment from images of older women having botox injections, of plastic surgery for both men and women, and of tanned older men with younger women on their arms. It feels important.

Worse, the opposite – the popular view of older bodies – has always been rather gross. 'Sans teeth,' was Shakespeare's view; 'wrinklies' is hardly a term of endearment, and everywhere we look there are pictures of wrinkles being ironed out by botox, flab being surgically removed, Fonda-esque body improvements by exercise and surgery.

It is easy to be puritanical about all this, but that is to ignore just how deeply ingrained our resistance is to this aspect of getting older. The broadcaster Joan Bakewell, once described as 'the thinking man's crumpet', wrote a thoughtful article about being over 70 in the *Guardian* in 2006, describing herself as 'vain by nature', and missing the admiration which no longer comes her way.[1]

'While old men are thought to be ruggedly attractive, old women are deemed to be beyond allure, devoid of sexual chemistry, a worn husk of their juicier former selves,' she wrote. 'I remain true to my inner self: I still enjoy clothes ... I still love high heels, have my hair tinted, watch my weight. I confront the mirror less often than I did, and when I do I make a harsh appraisal, and do my best with what's left.'

The publisher Diana Athill says something similar about the experience of ageing:

> The most obvious thing about moving into my seventies
> was the disappearance of what use to be the most
> important thing in life: I might not look, or even feel, all
> that old, but I had ceased to be a sexual being, a
> condition which had gone through several stages and had
> not always been a happy one, but which had always
> seemed central to my existence.[2]

Then out of the blue, at the end of 2005, a series of advertisements for Dove soap included a woman in her nineties, admittedly a model, advertising the soap as much younger women were doing. The point was being made that we have to love and respect our bodies, fat, thin, young or old. For many people, the image of a nearly naked woman of this age was deeply shocking. For others, it came as a welcome relief from the constant bombardment with images of young, thin, ditsy blondes, resplendent on the arms of men, the bonnets of cars, or simply wearing gorgeous clothes that are manifestly unsuitable for older women.

The other side of this debate is why we need to be quite so ashamed of our older bodies. Michele Hanson wrote about catching sight of herself (aged 60 plus) with horror in the mirror in the changing rooms in Marks & Spencer.[3] 'Of course I tried things on,' she wrote. 'But if you are a repulsive old crone, no garment can help you, so I sat down on my ghastly sagging bottom and wept.' Why does it have to be that way, at least so much?

The fear of wrinkles are such that those supermodels over 40, with their botox-smooth skin, risking cancer with their human growth hormone, prioritize their removal over almost everything else. It is almost as if there is a class divide: those who can afford it chop themselves and stitch themselves up again to make sure they look no older than 30; the rest of us wrinkle.

There is a very long way to go before women start accepting their wrinkles, but there are signs of something happening. There are new images of beauty and maturity as advertisers begin to wake up to the possibilities of the older market. The issue is being discussed more openly and, in July 2007, even *Vogue* celebrated 'ageless style'. The journalist Virginia Ironside, in her excellent book *No, I Don't Want To Join a Book Club*, set out a wonderful list of rules for how to dress after middle age, most of which were given to her by her mother.[4] They include:

1 Never wear white. It makes yellow teeth look yellower.
2 Always keep your upper arms covered. Those bits of flesh that hang down at the sides (known, apparently, as bingo wings) are hideous, and so are those strange rolls of flesh that appear between your underarms and your body.
3 Get a new bra every six months.
4 Don't disguise a lizardy neck with a scarf or polo-neck. They always look as if you have something to hide.

5 Never wear trousers after 50, unless they are ludicrously well cut and slinky, and never wear short skirts.
6 Make sure you possess and wear the most glamorous dressing gown in the world.

When a 56-year-old woman called Mary asked the Age Concern discussion website whether people should 'dress and live like the age I'm supposed to be?', she was overwhelmed by the response.[5] This came from much older women refusing to grow old 'gracefully', quoting Jenny Joseph's famous poem 'Warning' – 'When I am old I shall wear purple' – and wearing whatever they felt like.

With the emergence on magazine covers of powerful actresses in their sixties and seventies – Dames Helen Mirren and Judi Dench – celebrated for their style, it is clear that older women are now more fashionable. That should be some comfort for those who are more inclined to worry about whether they could fit into fashionable shoes.

But there is still a very long way to go. If the advertisers and the fashion magazines are beginning to shift, and the newspaper columnists are beginning to talk about it, that is important. But older people worry about it enormously, and those professionals whose job is to care for them later – and who make policy about their care – often have not the slightest idea that appearance is important to them at all.

The issue of what to wear and how to wear it remains hotly debated. What seems to unite older people I talked to was that it was important to do it with style and effort, because of the message that action gives to yourself and others that you remain an active human being. The business of appearance underpins the active role that older people play, and therefore helps them stay healthy and happy.

Work

I wrote at the beginning of the book about how much my mother wanted to go back to work when she was in her eighties. There is no doubt that older people wish to feel that they are active providers in the community, that they are a useful part of society, and that they are not a burden on others. It is the other side of keeping up appearances: older people have to protect their self-respect, not just by looking as if they are playing a useful role, but by actually playing one.

Of course, people manage being active providers better if they live in their own homes, and are mobile enough to get to family, friends and shops. They also have to be in reasonably good health, but that is not an absolute. Even if older people's health is getting worse, there are ways of making sure their quality of life holds up, or at least that it doesn't go down at the same speed. There are a range of technological advances that can keep people independent.

Productivity means different things to different people. So many of my discussions with older people make it clear how much they long to be back at work. This might be because they need to earn more money, but it is about more than just money. For many of them, it seems to be a sense of being of value. The more our society judges people by what they do, rather than by who they are, the more older people are going to want to go back to work. Of course they will.

The point is that even those who have run their own businesses, or been very senior in some major corporation, and who have all the money anyone could wish for, still need to be needed, and long to be asked to do something, however unlikely, that gives them a role. In the United States, where people retire later – if at all – this is sometimes provided by continuing to go to work, and often by getting a more and more senior-sounding title, even though the role is in fact less influential than the one the same person held in their forties. It is hugely important that this has happened: the people concerned feel valued, still have an office, a secretary and a role, and are often wheeled out at all sorts of occasions to do some glad handing or to look after more junior staff.

In fact, when the bank HSBC carried out a huge survey of 21,000 people on the subject in 2006, it showed that more than 70 per cent of people in countries such as Canada, the United States and Britain say they want to work into their old age.[6] Many of those who took part in the survey were clear that they wanted to work on their own terms, part-time or seasonally, with switches between periods of work and periods of leisure. Surprisingly, HSBC's advisor on retirement said he thought the British were the most positive in the world in their attitude towards working in retirement, perhaps because the pensions are so poor here that people simply have to think differently. Or perhaps because opportunities are finally emerging for older workers to work differently from earlier in their career, more flexibly, and with increased satisfaction.

If so, there is still a very long way to go. An ICM poll for the BBC's *Newsnight* programme in 2004 suggests that people are more than irritated at the discrimination against older workers. But there is a peculiar contradiction here. Only a few months earlier, when Lord Turner had published his pensions report, much of the media coverage had been about being 'forced' to work longer, to 67, 68 or 69. On the one hand, the polls suggest people want to work longer, albeit more flexibly; on the other hand, the commentators are telling us that people are resisting the idea.

The answer is that it depends what we mean by 'work'. It depends on what the work is, whether we feel we are being cheated out of a pension we have earned, and a retirement date, whether pensions will be clawed back if we are earning, whether we are allowed to be flexible about how we work, whether the jobs can be rewarding in older age and, perhaps most significantly, how much we can feel independent. If people are self-employed, then they might reasonably expect to carry on working because they have customers, the most natural thing in the world. Maybe others can reinvent themselves to become self-employed later in life in order to do something totally different and, of course, find the customers who want to buy.

The *Independent* columnist Hamish McRae suggested that, a generation from now, a quarter of the workforce will be self-employed, which will change the nature of the pensions debate completely.[7] The Turner proposals, and all the others, assumed that people are mainly employed by somebody else. But if McRae is right, then a large proportion of older people will be self-employed, carrying on working, perhaps less energetically than before, but possibly just as devotedly, and arguably with greater experience.

Some will be new self-starters, like Jacquie Lawson, of JacquieLawson.com, who became the market leader in online greeting card, at the age of 62.[8] After six weeks of trial and error, having taught herself how to do it using Macromedia Flash, she sent a Christmas card to various friends in 2000, and went to Australia. When she got back, there were some 1,600 messages from people all over the world who had seen it and wanted her to set up a website. She did, but it crashed under the strain of huge demand. So friends and relatives helped her set up her business, investing in higher-grade technology, and she became an instant success. Not everyone does so well, but Jacquie Lawson is a shining example of someone who wanted to keep going as she got older, and had some good ideas.

There are also moves to keep people employed beyond retirement age. Older employees are being encouraged to stay at work longer to prevent a 'dependency crisis'. That applies to both women and men, but women are more concentrated in poorer-paid and part-time jobs, so their financial provision for old age tends to be worse than men's – and they tend to live longer too. As a result, we are seeing women in the workforce to an increasing extent, especially amongst older age groups.

There are 1.5 million women in the workforce between the ages of 45 and 64, and some 113,000 over 65, when women's 'official' retirement age is still 60. For many of these women, the effects of working are wholly beneficial: more money, better mental health, better self-esteem and better social networks. A large body of evidence suggests that many women of all ages get much of their social support from colleagues at work, and this must be particularly true for women who have been widowed or whose children have moved away.

Official efforts

Despite a new official desire to keep people at work longer, and a plethora of initiatives to make sure that this happens, there are huge challenges in finding and keeping a job in later life, especially in areas of high unemployment, in the toughest regions or the toughest sectors. There is also real age discrimination. This is partly because of obsolete social protection schemes which means that older people get their earnings stopped to pay for their social support.

There is still a prevailing view that older workers are too costly and resistant to change. The Social Exclusion Unit of the Office of the Deputy Prime Minister reported in 2004 that the low level of older workers in jobs costs the economy between £19 and £31 billion a year in lost output and taxes, and increased welfare payments, not to mention all those skills lost to employers.[9] Yet nine out of ten older people believe that employers discriminate against them, and a quarter speak from experience. As many as ten per cent of companies refuse to employ anyone over 50.

The European Union is now resolved to do something about this, given the waste of resource so many older people not working represents. The idea of anonymous CVs certainly helps people from ethnic minorities, another group who are unfairly discriminated against in employment, but they are very little help to older workers, because a glance at the work history gives away the rough age of the applicant.

Some EU member states have tried to create incentives for employers to hire specific age groups by making them more attractive – that is to say, less protected – than the rest of the workforce. But this approach has not really helped either, though those countries which have a rather different approach, and a range of positive active ageing policies, are succeeding in attracting older workers. It works where working conditions are improved for everybody, with early retirement schemes being restricted to cases where major restructuring is inevitable, and where allowing part-time work to be combined with part-time pensions is the norm, so that people are not caught in a social benefit trap where it simply is not worth their while to work.

The European Union is worried about their ageing populations and falling birth rates. Japan is facing similar issues, and tackling them by paying grants to employers of older people and by other means of supporting older workers directly. The Japan Organization for Employment of the Elderly and Persons with Disabilities (JEED) does a huge amount of work trying to get older people into work, and they also work to police the new law which forces employers to take measures to keep people in work until at least 65.

JEED provides counselling and advice services on employing older people, and the measures – half of the costs of which are paid for by the government – include health management counselling, specialist advice services for re-employment, and much else besides. This is so far in advance of anything done in Europe that it seems amazing to us, and yet these are exactly the kinds of measures we need to see if older people are to be comfortable at work and not treated as slightly eccentric for continuing to want to be there. They are also working away at a long-term 'Project to Develop a Solid Foundation for a Society Where People Can Work Regardless of Their Age (The Age-free Project)', to find out what kind of systems would be needed so that anybody can work regardless of age.

But beyond the subsidies to companies that are making efforts in this direction, there is support for self-employment too. If three or more older people (aged 45 plus) have united to start an enterprise, and are themselves employing workers, they can get grants to pay their start-up costs. All this is serious stuff, and worth close examination if the UK, and Europe more widely, are to be anywhere in the same league in employing older staff.

What kind of work?

Thanks to a recent ESRC Report, *Older People's Experience of Paid Employment: Participation and Quality of Life*, by a team from Sheffield University, we know that 'the highest levels of well-being in any category were among those who were employed when over retirement age'.[10] But – and this is the most important finding – of all those who were employed, life satisfaction was highest among the part-timers, and lowest among those who were forced to carry on working because they needed the money. In other words, it is not just a question of whether one is employed, unemployed or retired, but whether one wants to be.

Whether people want to be employed depends on their finding work which suits them. So there really does need to be more room for part-time and flexible employment for older people, which many say is what they want. The 2003 Joseph Rowntree Foundation report *The Role of Flexible Employment for Older Workers* showed that the choice depends partly on who you are.[11]

Leaving work tends to be a positive choice for workers with other advantages – including those (especially men) who have been with their present employer for longer, and are therefore more likely to have accumulated savings and pension entitlements, and those who have paid off their mortgages. People with health problems are also inclined to leave work early, especially low-paid men. But 'early retirement' for them is more likely to mean they were unable to stay employed, rather than something they chose.

Self-employment offers the job quality most comparable to that enjoyed by permanent full-time employees. Temporary employment rates next in terms of job quality, although this is more the case for people on fixed-term contracts than for casual workers or agency temps. Part-time employment offers the poorest job quality among the three types of flexible employment, and yet it is extremely popular amongst many older people. Overall, women appear more successful than men in finding flexible jobs for positive reasons, but they often find that these jobs are poor quality, or extremely badly paid.

It is worse than that for many part-time older women workers, according to the report *Older Women, Work and Health* (Lesley Doyal and Sarah Payne).[12] Some of the supposedly 'light work' offered to women often leads to musculoskeletal disorders as a result of repetitive strain injury from keyboards or simply from having to move heavy loads which no one had recognized as being necessary. Take French train cleaners, for example. Doyal and Payne found their labour force was mixed, but only the women were allocated to cleaning the toilets, which was work that was dirty, physically demanding and required considerable technical skill. It involved travelling over 20 kilometres a day and maintaining uncomfortable postures, with a quarter of the time in a crouched position. It is hardly surprising that those women suffered from high rates of back pain and other problems and were often absent from work.

'Work is usually a healthier occupation for a 60-year-old white solicitor, for example,' says the report, 'who has a high degree of control over her working life and can buy domestic help if she needs it, than it is for a 60-year-old African Caribbean office cleaner, with little job security and a heavy domestic burden.'

Even our own community nurses, coming up for retirement at 55 with relatively generous pension settlements, show little sign of being lured back to work, even when they are told that they will be able to keep their full pension and earn on top, so desperate is the need for their skills and experience. So, despite all the evidence of older women gaining benefits from continuing to work, it is clear that for some women the thought of carrying on – perhaps because they are burnt out by what they have been doing, because they do not trust management, or because they have seen too many upheavals in organizational terms in recent years – just doesn't appeal very much.

So there is a paradox here, at least. Most research agrees that staying in work for women provides them with better social networks and keeps them healthy. Yet whether they actually want to work depends on a range of other factors, like flexibility, stress, respect, conditions and safety: the rate of slip, trip and fall injuries rises significantly with age for women, but not apparently for men. So we have to do more to prevent accidents, more to appreciate those women and what they do, and perhaps more too in those health professions where they are in short supply to give them control over their own work.

Age discrimination

The real question, behind all of these questions, is more fundamental. Why has government in the UK, and governments more generally, not made it easier to carry on working? Why have they only woken up to the need because they are frightened of the demographic time bomb? And why is there such a culture of retirement at 60 or 65, which clearly does not suit many people – especially when research shows that, if all the older people who wanted to work actually found jobs, they would generate economic output as high as £30 billion?

There are excellent economic reasons like this why society needs to make it easier to carry on working, but the real reason our governments have been so slow is probably the same reason employers have been so slow. They discount the skills and experience of older people, and cling to an increasing faith in those of the young.

'If the offices of the FTSE100's chief executives had a theme tune, it would be the refrain of Bob Dylan's 'My Back Pages': 'Ah, but I was so much older then, I'm younger than that now,' wrote *The Times'* then business editor James Harding, in 2007.[13] The average age of FTSE 100 chief executives had fallen by nine months to 52 over the preceding five years and, at the beginning of 2007, there were more top British chief executives in their 30s than in their 60s.

Strangely enough, Europe is going against the trend in the USA and Asia in this respect, where average ages are rising. It is almost as if, as power is passed to an ever younger age group, they feel that much more uncomfortable about the voice of experience. 'Corporate Britain is squandering experience, driving out good people ... when they are in their prime,' wrote Harding. 'There is too much age concern in the executive suite.'

There is such double-think about all this, when 90 per cent of us think old people should be cherished and 60 per cent think the elderly enrich our cultural life. 'Oh really?' said the columnist Janet Street-Porter. 'If that is the case, how come we don't take the time and trouble to know any of these national treasures? Half those under 24 who were surveyed didn't know anyone over 70, and vice versa. If old people are so supersonic, how come the country is full of homes where ageing relatives have been parked out of sight?'[14]

Of all those organizations most active in their age discrimination, the most obvious are the broadcasters. The BBC ran into trouble for dropping Nick Ross from his own *Crimewatch* programme, which he started presenting in 1984, at the age of 59. They had already had negative comment about dropping the newsreader, Moira Stuart, on the basis she looked too old. Joan Bakewell was dropped from a TV show called *Rant* on Channel 5 because she was not within 'their audience demographic'. Too old, it seems. Why is it that broadcasters are so dismally knee-jerk in their pursuit of younger viewers and listeners, forgetting that Terry Wogan still pulls in a huge audience at well over sixty, and that the oldies' market is growing, not shrinking?

Those who depend on broadcast coverage are especially vulnerable as Sir Menzies Campbell discovered in 2007. But those who need no broadcast coverage are still heaved out of their jobs at 65. With new age discrimination legislation in place, is it legal – let alone morally acceptable, which it plainly is not – to discriminate against older workers on the basis that the right to claim compensation for unfair dismissal and statutory redundancy pay stops at 65?

If the FTSE 100 companies are not setting an example, who will? But those at the opposite end of the debate are not setting an example either. A huge number of public sector workers believe they have the right – or at least they exercise this opportunity – to take early retirement at 55. Many people are forced to retire early, admittedly on pretty well near a full pension, because of reorganization after reorganization, especially in the NHS. But the idea that we can leave a job and get a full pension at 55 as a teacher, a community nurse, a hospital nurse, when society is crying out for more people with real experience to do these jobs, is absurd. Yet any attempt government makes to convince public sector workers to stay longer, to forego their very generous pension rights – which were once seen as a compensation for not earning so well when working, which is less true now – has been met with a truculent refusal to negotiate.

There must be a better way forward, given the evidence that many older people find life more satisfying if they are still working. The 55-year-old teachers, social workers and nurses might be persuaded to work to 60 or 65, or longer if possible, if they could get a six-month sabbatical on full pay at 55. Sabbaticals are good for people, whereas retirement seems less beneficial than people used to think. They could learn something new, travel, see people doing their kind of work somewhere where they do it quite differently, and then come back and work at least another three to five years. It would save the public purse considerably in terms of training new people who would also expect to retire at 55. It would keep very experienced people in the workforce. But for those who feel burned out by the constant changes, or just worn out with dealing with difficult, inattentive children in the classroom, it would refresh them and excite them.

Surely before we accept the public sector's refusal to work longer, despite the obvious need, as well as the benefits to the workers involved, we should try more of a carrot approach. Indeed, those older people who go on grown-up 'gap years' are obviously fulfilled by it, learn a lot, and have much to teach the rest of us, if only we would let them.

There is a proposal that older drivers should be given cognitive tests every five years to retain their driving licence, because studies have indicated that older drivers are more likely to be involved in accidents. At the moment motorists aged 70 or more have to report any medical condition which may affect their ability to drive. When this was first reported, the *Times* had an online debate, and some of the responses make appalling reading. 'The elderly are dangerous enough as pedestrians without letting them drive cars!' wrote Simon Moss of Kiev in the Ukraine. 'The cognitive tests ... look pretty ridiculous too. A five year old or a drunk could easily pass them. Wouldn't an eye text be more relevant? Or a test of reaction times? Or would that be more politically incorrect?'[15] Yet all the evidence suggests younger drivers cause far more accidents than older ones, though clearly we could all agree that older drivers with cognitive or visual impairments should not be driving. The point is not the age, it's the condition that counts.

Volunteering

Huge numbers of volunteers, in all sorts of sectors of society, are in fact 'older people'. About a third of us in Britain volunteer regularly, though some of that may be extremely infrequently. Many organizations rely heavily on older people to make their activities work, whether it is helping schools with reading or helping in care homes – in some care homes the average age of the volunteers is higher than that of the residents. Large numbers of older people volunteer at the National Trust – I met a National Trust volunteer in her eighties who had become one of the country's leading experts in eighteenth-century furniture polishing. There are older volunteers in hospitals, working on anything from shopping trolleys to libraries, from showing people around to helping people who have mobility difficulties.

There has been a range of government schemes to encourage older people into volunteering, from the Experience Corps, which has sadly gone into abeyance, more or less, and was perceived to be unsuccessful by government, to Volunteering in the Third Age (VITA), and enormously effective operations run by charities like Help the Aged, Age Concern and CSV. But government has been obsessed with younger people volunteering – perhaps understandably – and has therefore mistakenly failed to keep a focus on older people becoming volunteers. The government can't tell anyone, young or old, what to do, but financial support for older people volunteering – and organizing volunteering doesn't come free – makes a huge difference to how older people feel, and to what they provide for the wider population. It also means they require less healthcare and general support if they are being active and feel useful.

The major focus of the government agenda on volunteering is on younger people, and particular groups of socially excluded people, those without educational qualifications, or with disabilities and long-term life-limiting illnesses, and members of black and minority ethnic communities, so older people do not always figure. Yet their contribution is vast: the VITA project's final report in 2007 looked at 477 organizations, involving a total of 1.3 million volunteers, two thirds of them over 50.[16] Older people are also disproportionately involved in the delivery of care to other older people.

One of the reasons they do it is to give them a reason for getting out of bed in the morning. The other benefits to the volunteers are obvious: enjoyment, health, a structure for the day, active participation in local communities, increased confidence and new experiences. The organizations that use them also gain, and so does society, from their long experience and skills, the ability to make connections between services and their users.

Take Roger Withers, for example.[17] He spends his time as a befriender at a local day centre at the age of 81 and eleven years after the death of his wife. Or Peggy Crudace, 85, who lives in a high rise block in Newcastle, which has within it a community flat jointly owned by social services and Community Service Volunteers. Peggy's 'commitment to involving people is one of the reasons the community flat is so successful. When she is not acting as treasurer, and taking care of the book-keeping, she is helping with the lunches, baking cakes, buns and tarts, organizing raffles, going to art classes, making decorated birthday and Christmas cards and even abseiling when she has the chance.'[18]

Or Ted Howell, 80, who was told by his wife who was already volunteering as a befriender 'not to be a slouch'. He takes people to hospital in wheelchairs, takes them shopping or to the hairdresser, and does anything else with them they want. Like so many, Ted is downbeat about what he does: 'It drives me out of bed ... it can be a pain in the backside,' he says. 'But it gets me to meet some very nice people.'

WRVS, well known for its work with older people, has suggested that we designate Christmas Day as 'Independence Day' for older people, in their honour, and, second, that we use the 3.5 million years of experience WRVS's own volunteers have between them to help others have a stress-free Christmas. To do that, they set up WiseLine at Christmas 2007, by both phone and email, to advise on everything from keeping the peace in families to present buying, cooking for a variety of different diets to solving the mysteries of fairy lights that do not function.

In their press pack, they highlighted a Liverpool volunteer called Maria who suggested having diversions at hand when tempers look as if they might get heated, and Shirley from Devon, 72, who has volunteered for 18 years and has just stopped running the lunch club which feeds up to 100 people each week – including people whom the local GPs beg them to take on because of loneliness, depression and simply a lack of things to do. And they do Christmas lunch as well.

But her most important point was about how you can still function as you get older:

> When it comes to ageing, I think some people think that the brain stops when the legs don't work so well, but if people get out and stay active, it keeps them engaged. People in their eighties can use email. One of our ladies was given a laptop by her grandson for her 90th. She went to computer classes and used it to email him in Australia, and to tell me when she could not attend or start her car![19]

These are not isolated stories. The truth is that, both in formal volunteering and in the enormous effort that individual volunteers make to help neighbours on a regular basis, old people are keeping the wheels of the community running. They are doing so even when they are frail and disabled themselves.

Barriers to volunteering

In some ways, the situation with older volunteers is the mirror image of older people in employment. They volunteer in overwhelming numbers and their contribution to society is huge and irreplaceable. But there are still barriers nonetheless, certainly according to 2006 research for VITA and Volunteering England by Colin Rochester and Brian Thomas.[20] Some are about the sometimes forbidding image of volunteering, and having the confidence to put yourself forward. Some are practical barriers, such as transport, particularly for poorer or disabled people. There are bureaucratic barriers related to the prevailing risk-averse official culture. There are barriers because of jargon and technology.

Insurance is one area which simply has to be tackled. Where formal volunteer networks turn people away simply because of their age, it is often because this has been stipulated by an insurance company. This is, in itself, a terrible injustice – not just to the individuals who are sent home to moulder, but to all those people they were able and willing to help. If somebody is fit and able to make a contribution, it cannot be beyond the wit of society to insist that they should be allowed to do so.

Inter-generational volunteering

The stories of much older people volunteering are heart-warming, but there may also be opportunities here that are being missed. The first of these is meeting the urgent need for inter-generational volunteering.

Some of this is happening already. Johanna Atkinson, 93, is helping children with reading but also telling them about her wartime experiences.[21] Iris Denny, 83, helps 5–6 year olds and 9–10 year olds with their numeracy. Judith Cohen, 80, helps young children to read and says: 'It makes me learn patience and humour in order to listen to slow readers.' Inter-generational volunteering works and gives pleasure all round. But, compared to the widespread need, it is still a drop in the ocean. Some children never meet anyone older than their parents; others never meet anyone with any time. Older children badly need the time and experience that older people have, not always as mentors, often just as surrogate grandparents.

So far, the brave effort going into organizing these inter-generational links is on a much smaller scale than it needs to be to make it mainstream, and it should be a central task of the education system to reach out and set them up. That has to go into the manifesto.

Humanizing public services

There is already a great deal of volunteering in public services: every government department uses volunteers somewhere in their wider organization, even the Ministry of Defence. A great deal of it is also carried out by older people. The work they do, especially in hospitals and the health service, is absolutely vital, both to the people who receive their help and to the people doing the volunteering.

When the first time bank in the USA began in 1986, run by the Elderplan health insurance company in Brooklyn, it was designed to encourage clients to volunteer to support older people in their own homes. But the real health impact was recorded for those who were doing the volunteering, to such an extent that those taking part were able to pay 25 per cent of their premiums using the credits they earned to recognize their voluntary efforts.[22]

But even without this impact on the lives of helpers and helped, there is another aspect which, even if it was the only justification, would by itself justify the massive expansion of volunteering by older people in public services. They humanize the way those institutions work.

When my uncle eventually died, in the hospital which really understood and respected his needs and treated him like a human being, there were volunteers everywhere. In contrast, there was barely a volunteer to be seen in the hospital which treated him like an object, although it was very well staffed. At a time when public services are becoming more technocratic, where the crucial relationships at the heart of their objectives are increasingly discounted, volunteers can and do make all the difference. In wards where older patients might otherwise be mistreated or ignored, older volunteers provide the eyes and ears that we need. They are also able to carry out work alongside professionals that professionals can never do themselves, like befriending. If this was embedded more deeply inside services it would, as Elizabeth Hoodless of CSV puts it, 'broaden and deepen' what public services are able to achieve.

What is true on hospital wards can also be true in schools, in parks, or simply keeping an eye open for how rubbish is collected in the streets. In all these, older volunteers can be a critical part of making them work effectively and humanely. But we need more effective ways of drawing in and using older volunteers, to make their presence at the very heart of our public services an absolutely core aspect of what they do.

Call to arms

When the first, fraught debate took place in Parliament extending detention without trial for terrorist suspects beyond the current 28 days, the House of Lords was the epicentre of the argument. Even without the hereditary peers, many members of the House of Lords are extremely old. I remember, on the night of the debate, some quite old men and women hobbling in, settling down to sleep on the floor of the library or in some other corner, and waking to vote every four or five hours.

By the end of the next 24 hours the legislation had been defeated. But I remember hearing several of those peers say: 'I went through the war,' or something similar. 'If Tony Blair thinks he can get shot of me, he'll have to think again.'

It made me realize how much society is losing out by forcing other people of similar ages out of work, whether they are capable or not. These elderly peers weren't having it: they rose to the occasion and took responsibility, and did so effectively. If they can do it, why are we stopping other people from doing it? Even the staff at the House of Lords have to retire at 65. So a key piece of our manifesto is that the government should look again at age discrimination.

- **People who are capable of carrying out a useful working role should be allowed to do so, no matter how old they are. It is time for age discrimination legislation to ban compulsory retirement ages.** The government should never have listened to the CBI when they rejected the idea of making the retirement age more flexible. Of course it is easier for human resources departments if people have a set retirement age of 60 or 65. Then they don't have to worry about assessing people's capabilities as they grow older. But that is not a good enough reason to justify the pain and ill health caused by forcing capable people into retirement, not to mention the sheer waste of their skills and knowledge. In particular, the manifesto should include demands to:

- **Prevent insurers discriminating on the grounds of age.** It is outrageous that capable older people are turfed out of their useful voluntary jobs for no other reason than that the insurance does not cover them. If they are capable of doing the job, then it is an appalling waste of badly needed skills for them to be weeded out. If they need to drive as part of the task, then they will clearly need to be checked periodically. But that is not enough reason for the community to lose their experience prematurely.

- **An end to the virtual ban on older people in frontline politics, women's magazines or television.** There has been a collective embarrassment about older women on the front of magazines, older political leaders and certainly about older TV presenters – even very slightly older ones. It is inhuman, wasteful and ignorant for this to continue, and no leader and manager should allow their organization to be caught displaying this youthful fear of age and experience.

- **New ways of organizing mutual support through local volunteering.** If older people feel the need for a role – and they do – there is no reason, apart for the economic one, why that has to be paid. Voluntary roles provide a similar kind of recognition, and equal opportunities for social contact and meeting people. A great deal of this goes on already, but there needs to be much more if we are going to provide the kind of social care an ageing population requires. It does not have to be useful in the strictly utilitarian sense, but it does have to be useful to the person who does it. And, as the National Trust does so well, it has to have recognition and status.

- **A massive opening up of public services by inviting in tens of thousands of older volunteers.** They will be the driving force that humanizes them, makes them effective and making sure that older recipients of care get the kind of humane service that they deserve. The way this can be done is to expect former hospital patients, for example, to play their part after they have been discharged, as part of a wider support network, checking up on patients who have been discharged, or engaged in other vital forms of outreach. What can be done in the NHS can be applied to other public services too, especially if the role of health centres and schools – even perhaps police stations – could be expanded to reach out into the local community and match surrogate grandparents with younger families and children who need them.

Chapter 3

Don't take my pride away

End begging for entitlements

We've been together now for forty years,
And it don't seem a day too much.

Opening lines of the popular song 'My Old Dutch', sung at the poorhouse gates where the performer is about to be separated permanently from his wife

While I don't have a problem getting out of the house, it's hard to find somewhere affordable to go. The cost determines what you can do. I'd like to go out more but I can't afford to. If I can't afford something, I just don't have it. Things aren't always easy, but you get through. I'm not defeatist – I can cope with most things ... The only thing I can't cope with is missing the wife.

Gerald Williams, 70s, quoted in Help the Aged Spotlight report

It is a good quarter century ago since I first got a wake-up call about some of the difficulties older people have with money, but it still feels shocking even now. I was a rabbi in Streatham at the time, and there was an older woman whom I came to know, who had been pretty confident and adept at making the benefits system work when I first knew her. Then she had a particularly nasty episode of mental illness, and when she had recovered she found enormous difficulty summoning up the gutsiness she needed to deal with the benefits office. She couldn't bear to go there by herself, so I went with her as her rabbi. As extra comfort, she also brought along her dog.

The dog was the first problem: the benefits staff were very difficult about her bringing it in. But there then followed the most extraordinary, frustrating and undignified interview. The benefits officer kept asking her for evidence to prove who she was. This was particularly peculiar because I was there to vouch for her, and I had brought my passport to prove who I was. But the real point was that not only was she well known to the system, but this benefits officer actually knew her.

They could see she was vulnerable, and knew she had been mentally ill, but they still gave her a really difficult interview. It was as if the benefits officers had been trained to be obstructive, and so it proved. In fact, when I complained about her treatment, I was told that this was normal practice.

It was also deeply unkind. It had taken a great deal of guts to go to the benefits office in the first place after what she had been through. I realized that the fact that she was old and vulnerable made it easier for them to behave like that. If that is not discrimination against the elderly, I don't know what is.

In the years since then, I have been struck by the huge difference between benefits offices. There are those that make an effort to reach out to older people and make sure they get any money they are entitled to, and there are those which – if they don't actually bully older claimants – take advantage of their reluctance to be supplicants to a complex and aggressive bureaucracy.

Let's not pretend that money is a problem for all older people. Many of them are extremely wealthy. But my time as a rabbi, and more recently chairing an NHS trust, has made me realize how many older people have real difficulty claiming what they are entitled to. They don't want to beg, so they don't try. The result is that, for those older people who are short of money, their financial problems are seriously exacerbated. There is a similar exacerbation of other problems in old age, like poor housing, for the same reason. That is how so many older people end up much more seriously impoverished than those around them.

Take the case of James Purvis, then 68, who featured in the series of articles written by the investigative journalist Nick Davies in the *Guardian* in 2005.[1] Mr Purvis lived in King's Cross, in a small, dark, damp flat – so much of the poverty of older people is related to housing problems – with a 'thin skin of mould ... on some of his furniture'. He lived alone, seeing few people, but had one pleasure: he travelled around London on his free bus pass, taking photographs.

He could not afford to take many photographs on his pension – just one roll of 35 photos a week – because he had to pay Jessops £7.99 to get each one processed. He made it a rule never to spend more than £5 a week on gas – he lives on his state pension – so, in the winter, he often stayed in bed for much of the day, and he only spent £5 a week on electricity, using the microwave his daughter gave him to keep the costs down on cooking food.

'Mr Purvis has cut down on eating,' wrote Nick Davies. 'Like many older people, there are other things he needs or wants out of not very much money, and food does not come high up the list.' It is no surprise that malnutrition amongst older people is common.

Indeed, the European Nutrition for Health Alliance argued in 2005 that poverty is probably the greatest social cause of malnutrition, combined with loneliness and social isolation, and the story of Mr Purvis fits this combination of categories perfectly.

His wife went back to Newcastle some 20 years earlier and he sometimes likes to hear voices that do not come from the television. Like many older men whose relationships have broken down, he also feels a bit of a failure, though he sees his daughter most weeks. But this is a common story of the absence of love, the absence of money to do the things he would like to do, and the recognition that – as he gets older and poorer, and costs of housing and gas and electricity go up – he will have to give up the one thing he really likes doing, his photography.

'He thinks it's a bit of a joke really, the idea of him sitting in this little flat all day, with the smell of damp and the curtains drawn,' wrote Davies. 'If there is no other way to make ends meet, he will just have to give up the photography and make the most of life alone.'

The story of Mr Purvis is one about a man who, though retired, does actually have a passion in life, which he is all but prevented from exercising because he is living in such poverty. Poverty and old age were such companions in debate a century ago, when the commission on the poor laws was first building a consensus for the first old age pension, that it was hard to discuss them apart, with the tragic separation of couples at the poorhouse door. The fact that we have had state pensions, however inadequate, for a century since then means that they no longer have to go together in quite the same way. As we shall see, many older people are quite well off these days.

Any book on old age must cover the question of money, but I am not going to write in detail about pensions, because it is a hugely vexed issue, and I am no expert. Pensions deserve a book of their own, and there are many of those already. Even so, money, its absence, and concern about it, are all key to any consideration of what old age can and should be like. It also looks as though our attitude to money in old age needs a great deal of re-examination. Whatever middle-aged people feel now, there is no doubt that younger people are feeling concerned that they will have to pay for their own pensions and their parents' pensions too.

These are important considerations when it comes to practical politics. People resent having to pay for long-term care in old age, and having to sell their home in order to do so, but the cost of the state bearing the entire amount might just be too great politically. Younger people would object. The politics of dividing the national cake is beyond the scope of this book too, so this chapter will simply look at some of the outstanding financial issues facing older people, and some of the things we might be able to do about them if we are really creating a manifesto for old age.

Poverty

Before we look too closely at the issue of poverty in old age, we ought to be honest with ourselves about how much richer, relatively speaking, older people have become over the last generation. The average net income of all pensioners (the technical term for older people, though not all actually get pensions) grew by 63 per cent in real terms between 1979 and 1996/7. During the same period, the average earnings in the whole economy grew by 36 per cent, which suggests an astonishing rise for older people, admittedly from a very low base.

The image of the poor pensioner was not inaccurate at the end of the 1970s, but the trend has been moving in the right direction. Older people's average income has grown even faster than earnings over the last ten years. The net income for pensioner units grew by 29 per cent between 1996/7 and 2005/6, whilst average earnings have risen by a mere 16 per cent in real terms over the same period, just over half the rate for older people. There have been substantial increases in incomes from occupational pensions, investments and benefits over the last 25 years. Also, average net income after housing costs has risen faster than the net income before housing costs are included, and this is at least partly because so many more older people own their own homes. Some two thirds of households headed by pensioners are owned outright.

Confusion about money

As I found when I was working on my last book, *The Moral State We're In*, poverty may not be as much of an issue for older people as it was, though there are still some appalling examples. But these are often more to do with not being able to think properly about money, and manage the daily administration and bill paying we all have to do, than with actual lack of cash.

The shocking Christmas story of 2003 was about an elderly couple living in London, in the same house for 63 years, who had died respectively at 89 (the man, of emphysema and hypothermia) and 86 (his wife, of a heart attack).[2] This was not the surprise. The problem was that their gas supply had been cut off because the bill had not been paid. Yet there was £1,400 in cash in their home and a further £19,000 in a building society. This was not a case of poverty. What was happening to them was that they were finding it harder to cope, a nightmare that overtakes many older people and is feared by even more. Though they may well not have Alzheimer's disease or any other kind of dementia, at the very end of their lives they often find it hard to organize things and get their paperwork sorted, to catch up with the bills and the personal administration, and to keep their affairs in order.

In the case of this couple, British Gas had cut off their gas supply but not alerted the local social services, and excused themselves for this appalling oversight on the grounds of protecting their customers' privacy, because of the Data Protection Act. The Data Protection Act's Information Commissioner responded immediately that this was not correct, and 'there seems to have been some incompetence on the part of the energy company.' Yet the seriousness of the case lies in the fact that two perfectly innocent, old and frail people – just about coping with the vagaries of life in their own home – died because no one noticed that they were a bit confused.

Much of that confusion was about money. They may not have been poor, but managing money, or trusting someone else to do it for you when you can't do it yourself – particularly if you don't have children or other close relatives – is quite difficult. It is also a source of concern, and even fear, among many older people.

Real poverty

Despite these trends, real poverty is still an issue for many older people. Some 1.8 million older people are still living in poverty in England, according to Age Concern, and inequality amongst retired people is greater than amongst the working population.[3] The top fifth of pensioner couples have a retirement income averaging around £45,000 per annum, whilst a quarter of all pensioners live below the poverty line (£5,800 for a single person).

All this is further complicated by the fact that some £4.2 billion in possible benefits for older people go unclaimed. Age Concern England has been trying to persuade the public to do more to make sure older people they know claim the benefits they are entitled to.

After all, the Department for Work and Pensions is on record saying that no pensioner should be living on less than £119 a week. Yet a third of us are afraid that an older friend or relative is missing out on cash benefits, and almost half of pensioner households fail to claim Council Tax Benefit, leaving almost £1.4 billion unclaimed. As many as 40 per cent of pensioners fail to take up their entitlement to Pension Credit, 47 per cent to Council Tax Benefit and 19 per cent to Housing Benefit.

Older people's charities, such as Age Concern and Help the Aged, already do a fair bit to alert older people and their families and friends to claim the benefits they are entitled to. But they could do much more, and this is where their polite approach to campaigning and providing help is less than useful. Many older people watch TV a great deal in the daytime, and a really angry television campaign might alert people to what they are entitled to. Giving them numbers to call and encouraging them to go to the Citizen's Advice Bureau – even taking part in the campaign – might also help. There was a high-profile launch of Age Concern's 'Your Rights' campaign, but we need to shame benefits officers into going out and finding older people who are not claiming. They are doing just this in some parts of the country; why can't they do it everywhere?

Fuel poverty

The poverty that older people are often particularly prone to is 'fuel poverty', not being able to afford proper heating. This is defined by the Faculty of Public Health as the situation where any household has to spend more than 10 per cent of its income on keeping warm. Older people need their houses to be warmer than younger people do, and often live in poorly insulated housing, or in their former family home, not having wished to move house, which is expensive to heat, particularly if they are living on their own. A total of 1.25 million pensioner households spend more than 10 per cent of their income on fuel.

There are government programmes to address this, but the £1.9 billion spent on winter fuel allowances may be a less than efficient way of tackling the problem, particularly as the need is so much greater for some than others.

Either way, fuel price rises are a major issue for many older people. Pam Greenhalgh, 65, who lives alone in Cheshire, admits she will 'skip a meal here or there or have hot drinks sometimes instead of a meal to make savings.[4] As long as I have my cup of tea, I don't care,' she adds stoically. Like many others, she uses pre-payment meters to make sure she has enough cash, but the costs are even higher that way. But she has to keep warm because she has arthritis ('my joints get stiff'), and if she is too cold she gets 'back in bed and keep warm under the duvet'.

This is not much of a life, and it goes some way to explain why 20,000 to 50,000 older people die each year as a result of the cold. Fuel poverty and energy efficiency have tended to be addressed separately in policy terms, but they are closely linked, especially for older people, because households containing people over 65 spend 80 per cent of their time at home – and this rises to over 90 per cent for people over 85. As Help the Aged puts it so beautifully: 'The state of older people's homes can be even more crucial to their general well-being than for younger age groups who spend more time away from home.'[5]

The oldest households are the most likely to lack central heating (22 per cent of those aged over 75 compared with 14 per cent in the general population). The worst-housed people are in the private rented sector, but these are mainly not older people. They tend to live in their own homes, but they still don't have the money – or don't use it – to improve their heating and insulation. And that, as we know, leads to poverty, and to unnecessary death.

Retirement income

So poverty has not completely gone away, but there are more complicated issues here. Older people spend less than younger people in general, and a greater proportion of what they spend is on food, housing and fuel. It isn't that older people can't afford more, but a combination of lifestyle and life capability, plus a nagging worry – felt by the wealthiest of old people – that the money might run out, makes them nervous about spending too much.

This worry gets focused on the issue of pensions, and of course people feel angry that pensions in the UK are not as high as in much of Europe, though many European countries are struggling to pay their pension bill. But there is also something strange about our determination to retire so early. I touched on the peculiarity of retiring early in the last chapter, but it is especially relevant here. Retiring when we are quite capable of working means that we become dependent supplicants to the state much earlier in our lives.

I am always being told that I sound like a middle-class person who enjoys her work. They ask if I would feel the same if my work were back-breaking physical labour, or mind-numbingly dull, but I'm not convinced. Fewer and fewer people, of whatever age, are involved in hard physical labour for a living these days, with the exception, perhaps, of nurses and care workers lifting older and disabled people. The majority of what was heavy manual work is increasingly mechanized, with a constant loss of jobs in those sorts of areas. But the new jobs are different, in service industries, computers, call centres or supermarkets. It can certainly be very dull stacking the shelves at a supermarket, but along with the relatively dull and repetitive work you get company, a sense of purpose – so highly rated by older people in how they describe healthy ageing – and some money.

Most of the examples of poverty in old age (see Gerald Williams at the head of this chapter) are also examples of extreme loneliness, exacerbated by a lack of funds. Perhaps working longer, and seeing work colleagues even a few hours a week, might help. The government tells us that we are going to have to work longer. Provided that work can be flexible, and that it is not compulsory, that is a very good thing, given our growing life expectancy.

If we do not work longer, then all the ghastly predictions about an ageing and increasingly uneven society, with the old depending on the middle aged for pensions and care, will come true. Working younger people will have to pay heavily to support us as we live on and on. If we do not work, we will need to find some other ways of giving our lives a purpose. We will also have to provide most of the care for our generation ourselves, because the young will not put up with the costs of providing carers to do all manner of things, if we are not contributing ourselves.

We say we were promised care from cradle to grave, but the truth is that this only applies to those who are old now. It cannot apply to those of us in our fifties and sixties: we are living so much longer that the social contract will have to be rethought.

The demographic 'time bomb'

Some argue that all the fuss about an ageing society is being made by those who want to reduce the levels of publicly funded support for the old and vulnerable, and that view is perhaps best expressed by the author Phil Mullan in his excellent book, *The Imaginary Time Bomb: Why an Aging Population Is Not a Social Problem.*[6]

He argues that the preoccupation with ageing has little or nothing to do with demography in itself, but is much more to do – as it always has been – with ideology, in this case the curbing of the welfare state. He also argues – as does Frank Furedi in his excellent introduction – that the problematization of older people coincides with 'the tendency to marginalize the elderly from the labour market and from society at large'. The real problem, according to this argument, is not about whether there are enough younger people working to support a growing population of older people, but that older people still find it hard to find employment.

How true that is. In the last chapter I covered some of the injustice of turfing people out of work early, and it is true that the employment rate of older male workers declined sharply in the late 1970s and 1980s.[7] These rates have improved slightly in recent years, but they are still below the employment rates seen in the 1960s. But what is being argued here is that this is also the crux of the problem of income in old age: that it is the shortening of our period of working life that is causing the difficulties, in financial terms, for older people and for the taxpayers, rather than demography.

There is plenty of evidence to support this theory. The Chartered Institute of Personnel and Development (CIPD) surveyed its members, arguing that Europe's population would age faster than almost anywhere in the world, and found two out of every five workers felt they had been discriminated against on the basis of age.

Older workers in traditional firms, such as banking, and in the public sector, also find themselves being made redundant. Cynically, they think it is because their employers can save money as they are 'expensive' employees, with years of annual increments to be paid in their wage packet. In fact, employers save little by making them redundant or giving them 'early retirement'. But they do transfer their costs to a different heading on the balance sheet. Until a few years ago, this could be almost hidden. Now, with a scandal over early retirements in the public sector, the true cost of pensions has to be shown clearly. Even so, if employers want to get the head count down, older workers make them feel less guilty, and they are often the ones who are most expensive, with accumulated annual increments and pension rights.

But it is not just about employment. Mullan argues convincingly that the fear of the demographic time bomb, rather than its actuality, is what promotes insecurity and a lack of inter-generational trust. If younger people think that older people are using all the assets, they will be suspicious of older people. That in turn will lead to older people trusting the younger generation less when it comes to looking after them when they are frail and dependent. The net result of this is alienation between the generations, instead of a mutual recognition of the need to care for each other.

This is a vicious circle, and Mullan is on to something when he points to the fear of the demographic time bomb as an example of the dwindling supply of trust in each other in our society, and particularly between the generations. His view is supported, though rather differently expressed, by the Rowntree Foundation's 2004 report *From Welfare to Well-being*, about planning for an ageing society.[8] This argues that Britain is still locked into a traditional welfare rationing approach for people on low incomes, rather than a broader approach that applies to older people across all economic groups as citizens and consumers, and which draws on the private sector as partners.

This may not sound the same argument as Mullan's, but it is. The welfare rationing approach is partly based on a fear that the next generation down is not prepared to pay for whatever is needed, so the obvious answer – out of fear of what might happen in an age-ing society – is to keep provision low. Yet if we took a different view, because we will not have to pay for unlimited welfare dependency – though some people will always need substantial help – and real-ize that older people will actually use and pay for a variety of serv-ices, often provided by other older people, the level of trust would improve. The traditional fearful approach to welfare rationing might, finally, gradually begin to disappear.

Financial products

The Rowntree Foundation also argued for a comprehensive re-think about the legal and financial architecture underpinning income in retirement.[9] We have had some of that, with Adair Turner's pen-sions review, published in 2005, and largely accepted by govern-ment. That recommended a return to the earnings link, but government has delayed that return by a few years, driving down the real value of the old age pension. Despite that limited success, Rowntree wanted another look at people's earnings in retirement, and at new financial products, from either the private or the chari-table sectors.

There has been relatively little interest by older people them-selves in these products, but that might be changing. Older people are now more used to buying financial products, and they may be more open to products designed for them, such as equity release schemes to fund adaptations around older people's homes, for per-sonal care or to secure more disposable income. Rowntree was not sure about the reasons for the current slow take-up of such prod-ucts, and whether it 'relates to a lack of interest by older people, or, as the Task Group suspects, is more to do with current products not being attractive enough for older people to purchase'.

One of the problems is that people are afraid, if they buy equity release products, they will lose out on means-tested benefits. The Rowntree report urged the financial services sector to develop a simple equity release product to help older people on low to medium incomes pay for low-level domiciliary care, and other services to support their quality of life. They also called for equity release products for properties of a much lower value than at present, and long-term insurance products which encourage older people to regain daily living skills, so that they no longer need the product on a long-term basis.

An alternative is some form of insurance against long-term care needs, which also contains some kind of no-claims bonus, or premium holidays which will waive the regular premiums if the customer has not claimed on the insurance because he or she had got better or had been successfully rehabilitated. It will be a small encouragement to people to try for rehabilitation and to go back home again, rather than go straight from hospital to a nursing home, and never emerge again.

State pensions

The third area where there is urgent need for a rethink is about when old age is perceived to start. As I said in the last chapter, we have to think differently about this: I am a member of the House of Lords, a place where many of my colleagues are only getting into their stride at the time that most people are being told they must retire. Even MPs in the House of Commons include formidable people like Gwyneth Dunwoody, 77, who says she will stand again at the next general election. We need to think of the trajectory of our lives differently, and not think of ourselves as being 'old' until we are largely unable to carry on working, and are limited to some extent by frailty and exhaustion.

But the point here is about when we should draw our pensions, and we have only recently come to assume we have the right to a period of good years before frailty on state support. When the NHS was invented, men did not tend to live long after their retirement age of 65. A few months or years was all they could expect. Trying to find what the life expectancy was of a man who retired in 1940 at 65, or a woman who retired in that year at 60, means looking at the life expectancy of a man born in 1875 and a woman born in 1880. If we take the 1946 National Insurance Act as the date to count from, we are looking at a birth date of 1881 for a man and 1886 for a woman. But life expectancy at birth is not the same as average age at death, which is actually more relevant. Most people will live longer than the 'average', as averages may include those who die in infancy.

Those averages gave a boy born in 1880 a life expectancy at birth of 43.7, and a girl of 47.2 years. If we take out the deaths in infancy, those retiring in 1951 could expect to live another 11 years. In 2005, this had risen to over 19 years. In fact, life expectancy of a 65 year old has risen by two to three months every year for the past twenty years, and there is no sign of the trend slackening off.

There is a famous story about the German Chancellor Otto von Bismarck, who was asked in the 1870s to set the pension age for government clerks. His response was to ask by what age most of them were dead. He was told this was 65, and thus the pension age was set. Seventy years later, when Sir William Beveridge outlined his vision for universal state pensions, average life expectancy at birth for British men was still only 66.[10]

In other words, the age of 60 for women and 65 for men was not originally a retirement age, as such. It was just a minimum pension age, after which everyone had the option of retiring and claiming a pension. In fact, Beveridge made it clear later that he thought older workers should stay in the job market. He saw higher pensions for deferred retirement as a way of keeping them in the workforce.

This didn't happen. The pension age was introduced by the Old Age and Widow's Pension Act 1940, which provided that the old age pension of ten shillings a week should be payable as from the age of 60, instead of 65, to an insured woman and to the wife of an insured man who has himself attained the age of 65. This addressed anomalies resulting from the 1925 Widows', Orphans' and Old Age Contributory Pensions Act. Then the National Insurance Act of 1946 allowed a pensioner with a wife under 60 to claim a dependant's allowance for her.

The original Old Age Pensions Act in 1908 had introduced means-tested pensions at a maximum of five shillings a week at the age of 70, paid through post offices to avoid the stigma of poor relief. You didn't have to be destitute. Then the Widows', Orphans' and Old Age Contributory Pensions Act 1925 provided the first national scheme of contributory pensions. Then, pensions were paid at the married couple rate when both spouses were over 65. This created a serious anomaly if the husband had been on unemployment benefit before – and getting an allowance for his wife – as he would have been worse off until his wife was also 65.

This is hardly unfamiliar, with all the various perverse incentives we see in our present benefits and pensions system now. There were then, as now, many anomalies and exceptions, with various people being entitled to pensions at various ages if they had been in voluntary schemes. The point is that there was a history behind the ages of 60 and 65 which makes them hardly relevant today. Paying a pension was not tied to a fixed age of retirement until after the Beveridge report in 1942.

Though the retirement age and the pension age are roughly delinked now, in that you can delay taking the old age pension after

65 for a certain number of years if you are still working, and can get extra payments calculated by actuaries to be 'fair' in terms of the cost of not claiming, there is more that could be done. If the government really wanted to encourage people to work longer, it would put more incentives into the system. If you delay claiming your pension, you would not only get a 'fair' extra payment but a bit on top as well, which would encourage people to work longer if they wanted. It would also make people feel better about themselves. It would usher in the possibility of varying retirement ages, making them more flexible, so that actual retirement would come when we couldn't work any more, and need more rest and support to carry on. The idea that because we have reached a particular birthday, we can now be put out to grass, or play golf all day, is strange and dated and needs to go.

The UK and other countries

The UK has always had a pensions system which provides a low level of pensions benefit, and which does not rise with contributions. Better-paid workers have always had to look to their employers or their own savings to get a reasonable level of replacement income in retirement. By contrast, most other Western European countries have state pensions that are higher in basic level and rise far more steeply with income levels than in the UK. As a result, the UK's state pension is far cheaper than that in most other European countries, with the exception of Ireland, which is very similar to the UK. That is why we have serious problems of pensioner poverty, and widespread means testing with all its attendant problems, while our European partners are facing problems of affordability and sustainability.

The recent changes to the UK pensions system following the Turner Commission will do nothing to change the overall design of the UK state pension system. The pension will stay mean. The delay in linking pensions to earnings will erode the value in real terms even further. Raising the pension age will cut its cost even further. The vestigial earnings-related elements of the system are being phased out. On the positive side, people will be entitled to full benefit after 30 years of work rather than 43, which will be particularly helpful to women.

But on the Continent, Italy's budget crisis makes pension reform especially pressing for the Italian government, while France and Germany have also announced ambitious plans to overhaul pensions. The huge stock market losses in 2007, the instability of the markets and the sub-prime mortgage crisis are also worrying people about the future value of their pensions.

Italy

Italy is where the crisis is at its sharpest. Their hitherto generous state pension scheme faces bankruptcy within the next decade unless some radical reforms are enacted soon. The state pension fund will shortly have to pay more out to retirees than it receives each year in contributions from an ever-decreasing national workforce. The governor of the Bank of Italy, Mario Draghi, put the problem bluntly:

> Today, the number of Italians over 60 is equivalent to 42 per cent of the working population ... That figure will reach 53 per cent by 2020. Unless the government gets its pension accounts quickly into order, young people entering the workforce today will have to pay contributions amounting to 127 per cent of their salaries over the next 15 years in order to receive the same benefits current pensioners receive.[11]

Italy is an extreme case of the effects of people retiring too early. The official retirement age at present for women is 55, for men 57, plus a minimum of 35 years of pension contributions. Under the latest reform scheme agreed by Prodi's centre-left coalition, the official retirement age will be progressively raised each year until 2014. But pension reform has been a major stumbling block for Italian governments for two decades, so it remains to be seen whether these changes will actually take place.

France

In France, pensions became a key issue in the 2007 election. The presidential victor, Nicolas Sarkozy, went on the campaign trail to Metz in eastern France, where he visited factories and former mines. The theme of his speech there was the same as the theme of all his speeches, that France had to work harder to earn more pay: 'If you think 53 makes you old enough to retire,' he yelled (he had himself just turned 53), 'then fine, go ahead and retire. But don't expect the state to pay for it.'[12]

Now in office, he is determined to overhaul France's generous welfare system and cut back on state pensions, which are crippling the country's finances. The state coffers are badly in the red. Public debt stands at 67 per cent, or five times its level in 1980. If you include gross pension liabilities, the debt rises to 120 per cent of GDP. One in four people are employed by the public sector and there are simply not enough people working to fund the pensions of those who are retired.

France also has one of the lowest labour rates in the world, with just 41 per cent of the adult population working and extremely few workers in the 55–65 age group still employed. And despite having the highest birth rate in Europe, France also faces the challenge of an ageing population. France's 2003 pension reform gave priority to extending people's working lives, to finance pensions in the long term. The retirement age is now 65 for certain groups and public sector workers must work for 40 years rather than 37.5 to qualify for full pension rights. But the unions are not likely to accept further change without protest. Previous attempts at reforming state workers' pensions have ended in mass strikes which have brought the country to a standstill and have toppled governments.

Germany

Germany has one of the lowest birth rates in Europe and, at the same time, people are living longer. In March 2007, the German parliament voted to raise the retirement age from 65 to 67 as part of a reform programme aimed at tackling rapid population ageing and spiralling pension costs. The government is hoping that by keeping people in jobs longer, they will be able to reduce the burden on the state pension fund.

But the decision has been heavily criticized by trade unions and groups representing Germany's 20 million pensioners and there was a series of demonstrations staged against the government's plans in Berlin and other German cities. The head of the DGB trade union federation, Michael Sommer, said the new law was tantamount to lowering retirement benefits.[13] Opposition politicians argued that the changes would lead to higher unemployment and increased pensioner poverty. Germany currently has one of the highest levels of public spending on pensions in the 30 countries of the OECD. The system provides a high level of cover, but it is widely believed to be unaffordable in the long term. Most Germans stop working, on average, at the age of 63. Critics say it is still too easy for workers to take early retirement and they claim that many companies encourage early retirement schemes.

Given growing concerns over the demographic time bomb, some pensioner groups have argued that people retiring now are receiving state pension benefits which are around 10 per cent less than they were in the past. According to some surveys, by 2030 one in three pensioners will not be able to make ends meet if they rely on their normal pension scheme.

Ireland

Ireland's property prices have soared over the past decade, and many Irish people saw bricks and mortar as a smart way of investing for their retirement. Buying houses overseas has also been hugely popular, as Ireland's booming economy has left many people with larger disposable incomes and opportunities to invest. Ireland's workforce has also grown rapidly over the past ten years or so, as the economy has grown, although – with a younger population than the EU average – Ireland may not have the immediate needs and worries of some European counterparts, where the workforce is closer to retirement.

At present the state pension for a worker who retires at 65 is about 200 euros (£135), though the government says it will raise that significantly over the next parliament. About half of the working population of 2 million people also have private or occupational pensions which will eventually top up what they are due from the state on retirement. Many of those are in public-sector jobs. In the private sector, one in three workers is putting something aside for later life in a private pension. Some commentators in Ireland believe that figure needs to rise significantly to ensure people's financial security.

Others

At the other end of the crisis scale, Hungary's population is ageing and dying fast, so that the country is set to lose eight per cent of its population between 2000 and 2025, according to the latest UN figures. Spain's pension system has been in a state of almost continuous reform since the transition to democracy during the late 1970s. In Denmark, the situation is made worse by strict immigration laws, which limit the number of foreign workers who come to Denmark and join the labour market, so the labour force stays older without the addition of younger immigrants. In 2006, their parliament, the Folketinget, passed a Welfare Agreement Act to increase the retirement age gradually from 65 to 67.

The UK debate

Meanwhile, in the UK, the biggest pension shake-up in 50 years is also happening gradually. The age at which we will be able to claim the state pension will rise gradually from 65 to 68 over the next three decades. In return for a delayed state pension, payments will be increased in line with average earnings rather than inflation. Generally earnings rise faster than prices so, in effect, the UK state pension will become more generous.

In an attempt to improve the state pension prospects of women – who often take time out of work to look after children – the number of years of National Insurance contributions it takes to earn a full state pension will be cut from 44 to 30. This will mean millions more people, mainly women, will be entitled to a full state pension. The government has also tried to tackle the issue of vanishing workplace pensions, as firms move to cut staff pensions. From 2012, workers who do not currently pay into a work pension will be automatically enrolled into a state-sponsored Personal Accounts pension scheme.

There has been a surprising degree of agreement over the UK government's plans for pensions. But it may not be enough, because the new pension settlement merely holds things as they are for now. The UK still has an ageing population and it will become difficult to pay for pensions and long-term care for the elderly if we don't work considerably more when we are older.

The literature on this subject is huge, and – even if this is no demographic time bomb, but a failure to let people work as they get older – there remains a problem. Peter Heller of the International Monetary Fund wrote a fierce study called *Who Will Pay?*, which makes salutary reading, and blames successive governments for their failure to 'take account of long-term risk'.[14] He argues that governments need better information systems and better ways of sharing information if they are to plan better, and he cites the UK, Australia and to some extent the United States as the few that take a longer-term view.

Not everyone agrees. Joe Harris, general secretary of the National Pensioners' Convention, says it is a myth that working longer is the only way to have a decent income in retirement.[15] But there is general agreement among commentators that something must change, from Adair Turner's recent report – urging us to work longer and save more – to Will Hutton of the Work Foundation.

Hutton says that 60 and 65 were never realistic as retirement ages, and looks ahead to a new future where work and retirement, work and leisure blur together. People will have mid-career sabbaticals in far greater numbers, as only the privileged few manage now, he says. They will build up credits for the work they have done, so that they can switch jobs and still take the sabbaticals. 'A growing proportion will work not just into their sixties but into their seventies,' he writes.

'Work will become more fluid with the boundaries between work and leisure, one job and another, and work and retirement ever more porous.'[16]

He is undoubtedly right, but then so was Stephen King in the *Independent* when the Turner Report on pensions was published, who said the bottom line in the debate was political, not economic. People will have to work longer, he said. 'Better, therefore, to have the debate now than wait until society's interests lie in milking the remaining workers dry.'[17]

The big political problem is that most British people say they don't want to work until they are 67. All the evidence suggests that they will have little choice in the matter, but there lies the great political challenge for sorting out the finances of everyone in their old age. And that's not the only problem. Given our relatively mean system, pensioner poverty will continue, despite many older people being very comfortably off, so we have to ask how the tax and benefit systems can be reformed to help. The Institute for Fiscal Studies carried out a study looking at these issues, and concluded that unless something was done 2.2 million pensioners living in poverty now would still be living in poverty in 2017–18.[18]

Bringing in the earnings link for the basic state pension in 2008 rather than 2012 would immediately help 100,000 poorer pensioners. Doing more about outreach to poor older people, so that people get the benefits they are entitled to, would help enormously as well. Full benefit take-up would reduce the present 2.2 million by 500,000 straight away. The last suggested remedy is the introduction of a basic universal state pension, paid irrespective of years at work. This would of course help enormously, but it is still very controversial, though it clearly benefits those women who can't match the new figure of 30 years in the workplace.

Call to arms

At the heart of this chapter is the question of whether the so-called demographic time bomb is real, or whether it is some kind of smoke-screen for undermining the welfare state. What seems to be the truth is that it is only a real threat if we believe we somehow have the right to stop working, and be paid to do so, at the relatively young ages of 60 and 65. If we want to generate the resources we need to allow people to look after themselves when they are really too old to work, then our manifesto is going to have to be clear where those resources are going to come from. The answer is that they will come from reaping the great benefits we will gain from working longer – differently perhaps, but definitely longer. That way lie self-respect, happiness, friends and also money.

But this idea of a demographic time bomb does damage even if it is not an accurate reflection of reality. It generates a kind of denial about the financial realities, and a fear which may also encourage us to put the plight of the very old out of our minds. The 'time bomb' myth is there: the Irish government has been using it to suggest new ways of paying for older people's care. The UK government used it to argue against the conclusions of the Royal Commission on Long-Term Care. The truth is that, even though there is a growing number of older people in society, the proportion who are truly frail and need enormous support has not changed dramatically. We have coped thus far and will probably cope again. The issue, even if the demographers tend to deny it, is *not* the increasing number of older people. It is how we treat them and what their lives are like that should concern us.

So the central demand for this part of the manifesto is one for all of us. **We need to give people incentives to work longer, increasing pensions for those who stay in work, and then focus**

pension resources at an earlier age on those who really are beginning to be unable to work at all. The idea that we can retire at 65, 60 or even 55 is not sustainable, and probably never has been. It is giving rise to fears of a 'demographic time bomb', which in turn is fuelling resentment of the needs of older people and a fear of them in society, which encourages us, at the very least, to turn a blind eye to their neglect and mistreatment. In particular, the manifesto needs a demand to:

- **End perks for those in their sixties who are perfectly capable of working.** It might be unpopular to say so, but I see no reason why people who are still working, who might be quite well off, should get free travel on public transport. Those resources are needed for those who are much older. There is an argument that free travel encourages older people to go out, but this is not an adequate reason for giving free bus passes to people in their sixties and seventies.

- **Integrate the tax and benefits systems to make sure pensions can provide for comfort, safety and warmth.** It goes almost without saying that pensions, when they are paid, need to be adequate, and for many people they are simply not. This is partly because people are expected to claim for a whole range of tiny pots of money to cover specific needs, so that those who are most in need are forced into being supplicants for hand-outs. If we integrated the tax and benefits systems, we would not just save money by abolishing one large government department, but the government could calculate what it owed to individuals, minus what those individuals owed in tax, and provide the proper sum, without forcing them to undergo the indignity of applying.

- **Get older people's charities to be angrier and more 'in your face' about the lack of advice and outreach on benefits – and put the squeeze on benefits officers.** Integrating the tax and benefits systems would mean that older people would automatically earn whatever benefits entitlements they are eligible for. But in the meantime, there needs to be a clear duty placed on the Benefits Agency to seek out older people and make sure they are getting what they are entitled to. Very large percentages of benefits are not taken up in old age, and this exacerbates poverty in old age. Without this outreach system, the state is in fact discriminating against older people, because it knows that they tend not to fight for their benefits. Benefits officers need to say to older people, 'You are entitled to this,' and some do. But much more could be done to make sure older people don't have to fill out the same form time and again, and that advice workers and local authority support workers and social workers, plus benefits staff, go out to isolated and vulnerable older people and help them fill in the forms. There are some wonderful schemes of this kind going on around the country already, but the picture is extremely patchy.

- **Launch a series of innovative financial products aimed at ordinary people,** which will allow them to save better for care needs, cash in the value of homes without undermining their eligibility for state support, and encourage them to get better after hospital visits – and to go home again – rather than sinking into inexorable decline. These products might also follow a new model in New York and ask people to pay partly in time, in mutual support for even older people, in return for care and support when they are themselves infirm.

Chapter 4

Don't trap me at home because there are no loos or seats

Reclaim the streets

Pity the poor pregnant shopper who needs frequent loo stops. Some shops might as well put up a sign in their window 'Incontinents Not Welcome' ... A woman's right to sit! A woman's right to pee! These may not have quite the same evocative power as the slogans of yore but as we get older, alas, they will.

Anne Karpf, *Guardian,* **25 March 2006**

As a park-keeper we used to go round and make sure there were no kids cycling. I know a lot of the kids that I nicked. They come down and bring their families on now.

Dave Pick, former park-keeper, in *Talking History,* **September 2001**

As she got older, my mother used to trip or fall over in the street with increasing regularity. Very often, this happened outside Belsize Park tube station, around the corner from where she lived in London. Usually, the greengrocer next door saw it happen, and rushed out, picked her up and dusted her down.

On one occasion, it was the dry cleaner who picked her up. She was bruised rather than badly hurt. But he also, very sweetly, took her coat, cleaned it, brought it back, wouldn't accept any money, and urged her to talk to the council, because she was the fourth person to fall in that precise place that day, on the same rocking paving stone.

That story reminded me, first of all, of the kindness of strangers, which is a key theme of this book. The truth is, whatever you read in the newspapers, that the vast majority of people are very caring and solicitous, and will always dash over to help an older person who has fallen over in the street. The other thing it reminded me about was how older people tend to see things. The dry cleaner understood that my mother minded about the fall, but she minded most about the state of her clothes. People hate falling over in the street, even when they are not too badly hurt, mainly because they get covered in muck and look like tramps. My mother said her coat came back better than it was when she first got it. I've still got it, in fact.

Later on, when she was in a wheelchair, my mother would only go out if she was pushed by her son-in-law or grandson. She refused to be pushed by a woman, which was incredibly irritating, and said something else – I assume – about keeping up appearances. She was in the wheelchair because she really couldn't manage otherwise, but she was confined to it faster because the falls made her increasingly fearful of going out on foot.

When we make it difficult, dangerous or particularly exhausting for older people to go out, we deny them full and fulfilling lives.

But we also hasten their decline, with all the extra expense in health and social care. We need to do everything we can to help older people stay active – to give them access to life – for both reasons. Yet, all too often, they are expected to pick their way through dangerous, litter-strewn parks, ride non-existent buses, or change trains using icy staircases, to spend mornings in town centres where there are no public toilets. It isn't exactly encouraging. This chapter looks at what happened to the promise of 'the good life' in later years of retirement, and what can be done about it.

It is important to understand what is actually happening to people from a biological and psychological perspective when they get older, since it is our bodies and minds – what happens to them and what we do with them – that are driving these changes. The biological processes of ageing are relatively well understood. So is the need to apply all that research to technology and design to improve the quality of life of older people. We also need to fund and coordinate research in all these areas. We know that.

But that is by no means enough. The problem is that policy-makers so often believe that, once the science and technology are understood, then that is somehow enough, when they still know so little about older people's quality of life and how to improve it. The Rowntree Foundation's 2004 report *From Welfare to Well-being* makes some important recommendations about promoting well-being among older people, rather than relying entirely on a biomechanical approach that is only really interested in measuring their sickness and health.[1] The objective of the report, said the authors, was to shift the focus from crisis support – important though that is – to much more pro-active support for older people to live full, active and independent lives for as long as possible.

That requires a radical rethink. Instead of focusing on a small percentage of the older population who might be very needy – and social services support is increasingly being targeted more and more at the very vulnerable, leaving early intervention completely out of the picture – the focus would have to be on prevention and health promotion.

Older people themselves want this too. It will help tackle the health inequalities in the older population. There is also growing evidence that an 'active ageing' approach is more cost-effective. Take T'ai Chi, for example. We know that gentle but regular sessions of T'ai Chi result in fewer falls.[2] They keep the body moving and protect people's sense of balance. But this isn't a technological intervention: the main hurdle is how to encourage older people actually to do it (by making it fun and rewarding it). The problems that need innovative solutions are social, and so are most of the issues at the heart of this chapter – how to help older people feel safer in streets that are dominated by young people, for example, and how to make them feel they belong in their own neighbourhoods. These may not be technological issues, and may not attract large sums of research funding as a result, but they are still absolutely vital. Because if active ageing, and having a good old age, are the name of the game, there are several major changes that need to happen in the way we live.

Public toilets

I remember listening to a Radio 4 health special on incontinence in 2006, and hearing a consultant urologist talking cheerfully about how women should not teach their daughters to go to the toilet just before going out ('Have you spent a penny?') as it teaches bad bladder habits. Apparently, it means their bladders are not wholly full before they need to urinate. I listened with rising irritation as I heard him argue that there were plenty of public conveniences, so it simply isn't a problem to find a toilet when you need one.

Of course it would be a man saying this. It is true that older men also need to urinate frequently in many cases, but it was quite clear that this man had simply never tried to find a toilet when he actually needed one. The extraordinary delusion which he was under is a kind of blindness to a problem that causes real distress to older women.

Because, really, there is little in society in the UK which is quite so unreliable as public toilets. A year ago, the National Consumer Council described them as a 'national shame'. The British Toilet Association – there is such a body – complained that our toilets used to be the envy of the world (so that's the BBC, the NHS, and our toilets) but are now often dirty or shut, with particularly bad provision for women, parents and children. Help the Aged also says that, along with the absence of chairs in shops, the disappearance of public toilets makes it hard, even impossible, for some older people to go out at all.[3]

This is not some minor issue. Public toilets are important for everyone, but they are particularly important for older people, who may have more limited mobility and may also need to use the toilet more frequently or with greater urgency than younger people. Those that remain open have usually also lost their traditional on-site attendant, which makes them less safe – or at least they seem so – which in turn allows the remaining toilets to be ruined by poor hygiene, vandalism, drug abuse and people using them as places to have sex.

It is so important to older people. Yet the provision and maintenance of toilets in public places is only at the discretion of local authorities. Under section 87 of the Public Health Act 1936, they have the power to provide public conveniences, but no duty to do so. For this reason, when parliamentary questions have been asked about the number of public toilets in each government region, you have to get the information from the commercial and industrial property data held by the Valuation Office Agency, not from the local authorities themselves.

So, even for parliamentarians, it is difficult to find out just what the situation is. But Birmingham Yardley MP John Hemming managed to get a breakdown, region by region, and found a decline everywhere, even between 2000 and 2004. An investigation by David Smith in The *Observer* in 2006 claimed that the number of public toilets in England and Wales had almost halved in the past decade – and that those that remain in town centres are 70:30 in favour of men.[4]

The British sense of humour is such that getting hot under the collar about toilets can make you look ridiculous. But it is a real injustice. Why is it that local authorities are rousing themselves to provide temporary loos for men to urinate late at night in London, but can't be bothered to provide loos for older women, knowing that this means that many of them can't go out? Why shouldn't they be allowed out late at night like everyone else? The reason this is happening is that we don't see the older people *not* going out, because they are not there. We see the men peeing in the street, so that is the problem that gets tackled.

There is another wilful blindness here. If we looked to see who was using the streets, especially later in the evening, we would find one large age group was missing. It is a serious injustice and a sign of faulty values, faulty perception and faulty ability to imagine and identify with other people.

Worse, many local authorities are pressing ahead with closure, assuming that somehow these responsibilities will be taken up by others. Solihull Council recently closed all six of its toilets in the town, advising residents to try the shopping centre, library or cinema. Clapham Junction, the busiest railway station in Europe, has one tiny toilet, which they were happy to close for refurbishment for months in 2005. As many as 14 million tourists visit London's South Bank each year, but there are no public toilets between Lambeth Bridge and Tate Modern.

It is hardly surprising that people are complaining about people urinating in the street – some older men are amongst the offenders. But a system which requires people to go to a restaurant or café, order a drink, and then use the toilet, simply makes the problem worse. In his engagingly frank autobiography describing his declining years, George Melly wrote about the time he was apprehended by a police constable while peeing against a wall in Shepherd's Bush. He explained that it was due to a medical problem. 'All right,' the young bobby told him. 'But next time, try not to choose the wall of a police station.'[5]

We are not alone in this problem. On a recent stay in the USA, I found that older women were to be found sitting in the waiting area – a sort of sitting-out area – outside the toilets (restrooms, as they say) in the department stores in Boston. These were sad places. Some presumably came because it was a good place to keep warm, with easy and rapid access to a toilet as the need arose. Others were there because younger family members were fed up with taking them to the toilet time after time. Better to leave granny or auntie outside the toilet, and come and collect her when it was time to go home. There were never enough chairs either.

When I went out with my mother, in the last five years of her life, and there were no seats, no benches and no public loos, it meant she was in real trouble. Why should we allow this to be the case?

The local government minister Phil Woolas did at least recognize there was a problem and suggested some ways forward.[6] These included a community toilet scheme, like the one in Richmond-on-Thames, where there is a deal between the council and local businesses. This gives people access to the businesses' toilet facilities in return for an annual contribution towards maintenance costs from the council. This must be a sensible way forward; it should not be beyond the wit of people to insist on this within local authorities. If McDonald's can provide loos, there is no reason why other businesses should not.

Woolas also suggested that it might be possible to include the provision of public toilets in planning requirements for new developments. He also suggested more mobile or temporary provision at night or peak times. Yet even where mobile toilets are made available by an enlightened local authority, as Kensington and Chelsea Borough Council do at Holland Park for their summer opera season, there is far too little provision for women, who take far longer than men.

Despite the old regulation that there should be no charge for the use of urinals (the 1936 Public Health Act again), the Greater London Authority (GLA) and Phil Woolas both suggest that most people would not mind paying for the use of suitable facilities, suggesting that a small charge would bring in enough revenue to start to make a difference. It would then be possible to staff the public toilets properly, to remove the fear that some older people have about using the public facilities that do exist, and to pay for a level of cleanliness and removal of drug dealing that would literally 'clean up' the provision.

But despite all the rhetoric, the problems remain. Of those who responded to Help the Aged's 2007 questionnaire *Nowhere to Go*, 78 per cent said that their local public toilets were closed when they needed them, and 79 per cent found that safety concerns made public toilets unappealing. Others said the hygiene was so bad that they were they afraid would get ill if they used them.[7]

This looks like it is one of those issues which will only be shifted by older people taking 'grey power' into their own hands. The Inverclyde Elderly Forum ran a successful campaign on public toilets, which is a case study on Help the Aged's campaigning website. It is also a story that is increasingly being taken up by local papers. The *Northwich Guardian* ran a piece branding the town centre's toilets 'a disgrace and an embarrassment' in June 2007. 'If this is the best that we can do, then God help us with tourists visiting our town,' said one local lorry driver. 'One look inside these toilets and they will be put off coming back to Northwich for life.'[8]

Anne Karpf called for a campaign (quoted at the beginning of this chapter) in the *Guardian*.[9] So did Rosemary Behan in *The Times*: decent public lavatories are a basic necessity for any civilized country, she wrote – describing the appalling toilets on a four-hour train journey, with no water, paper or soap, and train staff who told her she should have gone before getting on the train.[10] She said it was time for a Compulsory Provision of Clean Public Toilets Act.

This is a long-term campaign, but we are all going to have to take part in it. Otherwise we will carry on seeing old people, and frail people too, confined to home because they fear going out in case they are 'caught short'.

Public spaces

The website of the Royal Institute of British Architects (RIBA) describes a research project in the London Borough of Newham which is unexpectedly revolutionary:

*Using the format of an annotated map to make visible
and give value to the experience of old people within the
public realm, this project will foreground the experience
of ageing in public space by literally re-drawing the
London Borough of Newham through the experiences of
old people as they relate to the environment around them.
Organized as a participative mapping project, this
research will become a visible and tangible
documentation of the presence of old people in the public
realm and an invitation and challenge to architect
practitioners and theorists of public space alike to
engage with the desires and anxieties and day-to-day
experiences of old people in the public realm.*

The project may have been described in forbiddingly academic language, but the work itself was anything but. It was organized by an
engaging young architect called Sophie Handler, who walked
through Newham with an anonymous older companion to see it
afresh through the eyes of older people. The result was most extraordinary. In a slightly eccentric, semi-fictional style, Handler came up
with all sorts of ideas that should be amenable to production, if anyone were sufficiently interested to listen.[11]

For instance, walls are good to perch on and are often the same
height as seats in shoe shops. How difficult would it be to make
walls with a little more 'give' in them, to make them softer
than the present hard surface which many older people find
impossible. Or how about reclaiming the streets by having a 'tea
dance' in the park after it closes? Or even having tea dances on a
regular basis, something that happens at present once a week but
which is always under threat from lack of funding, as Handler
points out.

The mayor of Newham, Sir Robin Wales, recommended a series of tea dances around Newham as the declining older population's contribution to the Olympic effort, but Sophie Handler laughed scornfully at the prospect of 25,000 pensioners waltzing into the velodrome in three-figure steps: 'I suggest that what is needed is an Olympic size community hall instead: some place to keep dancing in.'[12]

While older people's needs in public space have a great deal in common with younger age groups – the need to feel safe, the need for appropriate facilities, the need to radically rethink how public spaces are used – there are many differences too. There are problems which affect all age groups, but older people most of all. Some problems are bad for everyone, but as the 2001 report of the Environment, Transport and Regional Affairs Select Committee put it, 'they are particularly awful for the disabled and elderly'.[13]

Sometimes there is a conflict of interest – or at least a difference in priority, often unacknowledged – between the specific needs of older people and other priorities. There are some areas where current thinking is encouraging developments that may be particularly beneficial for older people. But there are many more questions to be asked in order to promote policies on public spaces that serve the needs of older people better than at present.

Crime

Crime is the first of these, because older people often feel particularly vulnerable to crime, although it is well known that – for many types of crime – they are far less likely to be victims than young people. Even so, whether it is because they often live alone, or hear or move with more difficulty, the feeling of vulnerability outside is real, and that is often enough to deter older people from going out and being as active as they would like to be.

A number of initiatives have tried to tackle this. Safer Merthyr Tydfil won a Lottery Monitor Award in 2003 for their creation of the Homesafe burglary prevention initiative, which fits locks and gives advice about bogus callers, and tackles safety outside people's houses. Community safety wardens aim to improve the quality of life in residential areas by providing an additional uniformed presence on the streets, acting as the eyes and ears of the community, reporting environmental issues or maintenance problems to the council, visiting vulnerable residents and victims of crime to offer assistance and support, and taking referrals for the Homesafe scheme.

Various areas of Leicester and Nottingham have been piloting similar schemes. It is clear that older people like having street wardens, in the same way as they like having 'bobbies on the beat'. The extent to which crime is actually deterred, and the extent to which older people feel so much safer that they go out more and are increasingly active, benefiting their health, has not – as far as I can tell – been measured as yet. But there is evidence that older people really appreciate having wardens on the street.

CCTV

Older people are also more positive than other groups in society about closed circuit television (CCTV). This is bound to be controversial, because it brings into focus the conflict between privacy and civil liberties on the one hand, and potential gains in public safety and the greater use of public space on the other. There can also be conflicts of interest between the rights of different socially excluded groups.

If older people welcome CCTV, a lot of younger people feel threatened by it and feel driven out of space that they once regarded as 'theirs'. There are no easy answers to this dilemma, but the debate itself illustrates the need to have an ongoing public discussion about the impact of policy on public space, and to make sure that older people's views are actively sought and taken into account.

Then there is the issue of risk. A 2005 report by the Commission for Architecture and the Built Environment argues that the drive to minimize risk threatens the vibrancy of London's public spaces.[14] It is true that some of the risks may seem minimal to younger people, but broken or cracked paving stones or simply uneven surfaces are a real risk to frailer older people. In fact, the safety measures and items on the street that CABE might regard as ugly or unnecessary, such as benches, large signs and leaning posts, might be particularly useful to older people.

But there is a wider point about how the perception of risk and the fear of litigation – rather than the actual risk – mean that resources are diverted into avoiding being sued rather than making places safer. Alongside issues around public toilets, benches are a particularly emotive issue for older people – preferably benches with armrests and backs (as the London Borough of Richmond has already specified in its guidance, 'to assist the elderly'). What we have to work out is what is actually needed to make public spaces safe, and make them feel safe too, for older people as well as everyone else.

Even surfaces, benches and places to stop and lean, large-scale signs and bright lighting are vital. But some grab rails and other 'aids' to help the less able may be useless and unsightly, even though they may satisfy every local authority's desire to minimize the risk of being sued because of an accident which the council could conceivably be blamed for.

Parks and urban green spaces

Within living memory, many parks were the summertime place of choice for groups of older people to sit and chat, particularly for older men. This no longer seems to be the case. When the House of Commons Environment, Transport and Regional Affairs Committee looked at parks in 1998–9, they found that older people were actually under-represented. This was compared with younger age groups, but also – and this is more important – compared to how many older people lived in the surrounding areas.

Urban parks in the UK have in any case been in serious decline, with the increased privatization of public spaces and also a great deal more emphasis on indoor leisure facilities. But one reason people have not been using parks in the way they used to is that many of them have no park-keeper or other authority figure around. I used to walk to work through Regent's Park every day, and noticed how many gardeners and park staff there were, and are still. But even there, one of the best-kept parks in the country, with more staff than most, it can feel a bit threatening towards dusk, with drinkers sitting in the little shelters and springing out at unsuspecting walkers or runners just to surprise them. No wonder then that many older people no longer feel safe in Britain's parks, however lovely they are.

So our manifesto will have to reinvent the park-keepers, those mythic figures who inspired both fear and affection in children's book and cartoon films such as Nick Butterworth's *Percy the Park Keeper*.[15] Or it would have to, were it not for the fact that we may already be seeing the renaissance of the park-keeper. The benefit of a human presence in the parks to keep order and deter wrong-doers has been rediscovered. This is much to be welcomed, particularly by older people, and about time too: only a quarter of British parks have full-time rangers now. Council cutbacks in the 1980s, and a short-sighted failure to understand the importance of a responsible human figure, meant that park-keepers were often replaced by teams of workers who tended groups of parks, gardening and tidying up, rather than being responsible for just one.

'We want a return to old-fashioned public service values delivered by a new multi-skilled, 21st century workforce' wrote Julia Thrift, director of CABE Space, after their 2005 report *Parks Need a Parkforce*.[16] 'Some 33 million people use parks every year – it would be unthinkable to have a swimming pool without an attendant or a library without a librarian – why should our parks be any different?'

Park-keepers are also the focus of several local authority safety initiatives, like Lewisham's Visibly Safer campaign. English Heritage has produced a report on the history and function of the park-keeper in part, at least, to strengthen the move to return park-keepers.[17] But even now, the role of the park-keeper is mainly about parks security, inspection and maintenance. How difficult would it be to add a facilitation function to their traditional role: facilitating events and encouraging people into the park, both old and young?

For older people, this might mean running a scheme for volunteers to accompany them on walks in the park. Or it could mean providing milk-float-type buggies to carry older people across large areas of parks to where they, and their friends, like to sit or have a coffee. Other options might include loaning wheelchairs or self-drive buggies at the park gate, much as some shopping centres do in shopping malls. This is a new approach – and one where older people themselves could take the lead – but it could enable far more older people to make use of local parks, helped by paid park-keepers and, presumably, a voluntary organization run by older people for older people, which decided what services should be offered within the budget available.

Transport

Using public spaces often depends on access to transport. Transport has become a fashionable 'political' issue, and the different policy imperatives often conflict. There is a great deal of emphasis on accessible transport, with buses which can lower their deck to take on a wheelchair, and special wheelchair housing on the buses. Even so, the move towards greener towns and cities, with more emphasis on pedestrian areas and cycling, has met with a mixed reception amongst older people.

Obviously, it will benefit everyone in terms of reduced pollution. But while some older people may be keen walkers and cyclists, and may remain fit into extreme old age, for most others the reality is that they have difficulties getting around. They need motor transport of various kinds, alongside access to convenient parking either for themselves, if they are still driving or for whoever drives them to wherever they want to go. That can be at odds with alternative visions for transport planning and the design of neighbourhoods.

For example, a local authority might refuse planning permission for an extension to a hospital car park, in line with green transport policies. But this can reduce access for older people and, perversely, it can mean more demand for patient transport and ambulance services. Other potential conflicts of interest may include the need for older people to have comfortable seats in bus shelters, while those who provide such facilities may also want to deter street dwellers, street drinkers or crowds of young people from making regular use of them.

Older people also have different priorities for spending. Mending pavements and providing benches in the street may be more urgent than improving facilities for cyclists, even though some older people cycle. While many of the green campaigning organizations pay lip service to the needs of older and disabled people, many of their real priorities concentrate on the younger and more physically able members of society, especially the drive towards pedestrianization that simply removes area of towns and villages from access by older people if they can't walk or cycle.

Several years ago, the Scottish Executive produced an interesting report by researchers Julian Hine and Fiona Mitchell called *The Role of Transport in Social Exclusion in Urban Scotland.*[18] One of their findings is that excluded groups like older people are more likely to experience transport-related social exclusion, and have to rely much more heavily on walking, on public transport and on lifts from family, friends and neighbours. Those in lower-income groups also spend more on fares for public transport than those in higher-income groups, yet older people and people with health problems were more likely to find it difficult to use buses, taxis or to walk for at least ten minutes.

The good thing was that two thirds of respondents said their local bus service stop was less than three minutes' walk away, although service frequencies declined noticeably in the evenings and on Sundays. They were also well aware of community transport schemes, but didn't seem to use them much, which suggests that they don't provide what is needed by most older and housebound people.

The report also found that 44 per cent of respondents (across all age groups) felt their public transport travel was restricted because they were worried about their personal safety after dark. And when they weren't suffering from this 'fear-based exclusion', 17 per cent of them felt they were unable to get on vehicles easily or safely, something that is bound to affect older people disproportionately. Unless public transport is much more geared towards people who are slow, frail, and have difficulty with high steps – leaving aside whether they are wheelchair friendly – it is difficult to see how many older people will be able to use it at all.

So there are huge questions about the use of public transport by older people, and the response by those who design and run public transport systems is far from satisfactory. Yet older people, including the youngest older people, take delivery of their 'freedom passes' with pride, and seem to use them all the time. However, some 80 per cent of the older population does not take advantage of concessionary fares, particularly in rural areas where there are apparently other barriers in place, perhaps because buses are too infrequent to get to town and back reliably in a reasonable and convenient space of time.

Nor do these schemes deal with the numbers of older people for whom standard buses are simply not feasible. Claudia Botham and Tristan Lumley from New Philanthropy Capital point out that more flexible transport is required for quite a large proportion of older old people to get from home to a bus route, or simply to make the journey at all. Community transport can be wonderful, but it is extremely patchy.[19]

They point to more flexible community transport in other countries, such as in Sweden. In the west of Ireland there is a weekly rural transport system, picking older people up every week from their homes and taking them into the local town for the day, a meal and a health check, and then home. They don't regard that as very extraordinary. 'The wide level of geographical variation points to a need for sustained government intervention in this area to deliver better services for all,' argue Botham and Lumley. But nothing has yet been seen of that.

Shops, shopping centres and markets

The other public space essential to older people, and everyone else, is shops and shopping centres or malls. There has been an increasing trend towards out-of-town shopping centres, often requiring private transport to access them easily. Associated with this is an alleged decline in small shops. The received wisdom is that older people prefer small shops, although the research evidence for this is unclear. But clearly a combination of declining local high streets and declining public transport is bound to limit the choices of older people.

What we do know from the United States is that older people congregate in public space in malls, that they are advised to take their exercise in them, particularly in the depths of cold in the winter or the fiery heat of the summer where the air conditioning in the malls make them a comfortable place to be. We also know that the public space in the malls in the United States tends to be populated quite heavily by older people.

In the UK, accessibility to shopping centres is undoubtedly an issue, but older people may be just as likely as younger age groups to access competitive prices and a wide range of goods. Disabled access may also be better in newer developments than in old shops. Older people will increasingly continue the practice they had established earlier in life of shopping from home, and will use the internet for some of their shopping. Others will congregate in the old street markets, such as still exist, and they are part of the reason for the revival in street markets that is accompanying the much larger growth of farmers' markets in many cities and rural areas.

Despite all this, some older people still prefer small shops. They fulfil a wider purpose by providing regular and local social contact, and they are easy to get to. So we have to ask whether the big shopping malls do enough to welcome and cater for people who may not buy large items or shop in bulk, and whether they have the facilities (benches and chairs in shops) and the goods older people want. We also have to ask how small shops can survive if they can't compete on price with larger outlets and online shopping.

We need to look at ways of keeping local high streets viable, insisting to the Competition Commission that not all consumers are the same, but that those who might just be in the minority – like older people – have the right to have their choices defended too. We also need local authorities to work better with landlords to keep vital shops thriving, without leaving successful small shops high and dry facing burgeoning rent increases which threaten the long-term viability of the surrounding streets.

We also need new ways to help people with their shopping, which could either be commercial or co-operative. Shopping is one of those functions that time banks and other mutual support systems carry out very well, and these need to be encouraged in town centres as well as suburbs for just this kind of need.

Technology and telecare

In January 2006, the Department of Health claimed that the use of IT to monitor vulnerable people in their own homes was successfully helping growing numbers of elderly people escape residential care.[20] Nearly a third of elderly people getting intensive care now live independently at home. Intensive home care is defined as a package of care that provides an individual with more than ten hours' contact with care staff and six or more visits a week from social services, and the government wants to see at least a third of older people needing intensive support living at home by the end of 2008.

Some 65 local authorities in England have already overshot this target. About 280 people already received telecare by early 2006 in Newham alone, ranging from alarms and monitors to voice-activated light switches. This is hardly cheap: the most advanced telecare flats in Newham, in blocks of sheltered accommodation, contain sensors that detect movement, extremes of temperature, when the resident has got up from a chair or out of bed, or whether the bathroom has flooded. The inside of the front door has a 'bogus callers' button that residents can press if they think they are being visited by a distraction burglar. Each sensor communicates wirelessly, on the 869 megahertz frequency – the European standard for telecare devices – with an alarm device that phones an alert through to a control room.

In Scotland, West Lothian is one of the leading telecare local authorities, and they offer a core package of fire and flood alarms to all householders over the age of 60, arguing that universal free access offers a chance for people to familiarize themselves with the technology before they need greater support. But they can provide much more – fall detectors, bed or chair occupancy detectors, wandering alerts, epilepsy monitors, video door entry systems and automated door or window openers. West Lothian says telecare saves over them 3,200 hospital days each year by getting people home quicker or preventing admissions.

Despite the evidence in favour of telecare, enthusiasts say the technology is not yet being fully exploited. The director of IT for Newham argues that his biggest problem is persuading doctors to refer their patients for telecare because of what he calls 'understandable medical conservatism'. 'We're the new kid on the block; we're coming up with a radically different idea and naturally people are going to be cautious,' he says.

Nick Triggle of the BBC set out a vision of the future:

The year is 2030. Mrs Smith, aged 98, turns to her electronic companion to find out what medicine she should be taking. An automated voice tells her: 'You should take one of your statin tablets for your cholesterol.' It then says her supplies are getting low so she electronically orders more from the local pharmacist. Looking up at a screen on her dining room wall, she sees an outline of her daughter moving around at her home 150 miles away through a 'virtual frosted window'. Her daughter can also see her elderly mother, comforted in the knowledge that she knows she is up and about. Later in the morning, Mrs Smith uses her companion to have a video consultation with her doctor.[21]

The evidence from Newham and West Lothian suggests that this is not a fantasy. The way houses are designed and kitted out will alter dramatically as the population ages. In Bristol, a pilot project is under way using the companion, an easy-to-use computer system designed to help people shop and access health services electronically. The device was created by a team at Brunel University and presented at a CABE conference, and is in effect a scanner attached to a laptop. Users can scan food or health items from a brochure and the information is then sent electronically. Other features include a voice and text system to remind people to take medicine.

There are already over 1.5 million older and disabled people who have community alarms which hang around the neck and can link them up to emergency and medical services. These are very popular, particularly amongst people who live alone and are afraid that they will fall and be unable to get up again. Far more elaborate inventions are now on offer, such as the Possum Companion, which uses infrared technology to control a variety of home appliances, such as security on the door, access for door opening, loud speaking phones, nurse call, pagers, operating power sockets, opening curtains and blinds, and operating entertainment systems.

I imagine that for some technologically minded older people who are quite frail, they must be a godsend. It keeps them independent and can help reduce the sense of isolation. But for many older people, they might be too difficult to operate, a stage too far in technological advance. But there are other reasons why not everyone is convinced by the benefits of the telecare future. Roger Battersby, director of PRP architects, warned that it could 'propagate social isolation while it is facilitating care'. The idea that you can replace human contact with tele-surveillance is, to put it mildly, disturbing. It has something of the feel of the old solution to psychiatric hospitals and prisons, the old 'panopticon' concept, invented by Jeremy Bentham, where one person can survey large numbers of people from his vantage point, but they can't see each other.

It really is better for older people to go out if they can, rather than have remote surveillance at all times if they have to be housebound. Surveillance is no substitute for simpler things like installing a handrail, or getting a neighbour to come in regularly for a chat. Those policy-makers who believe technology is a solution by itself are not seeing the needs of older people clearly – as if an 'electronic companion' was somehow an adequate substitute for a real companion, or as if only seeing people on screen was somehow a reasonable substitute for actually meeting them. There are American gurus of virtual intelligence who see no difference. They are quite wrong: people need human contact, and telecare – however sophisticated – does not fulfil this need.

Nor does telecare cope with those whose vision is poor, or with power cuts or when the technology simply does not work. If it is used to make sure people are safe and moving about, or even to check their heart rate and blood pressure, it could clearly be useful, although it is hard to see how 'care' can be delivered remotely, without direct human involvement. The point here is not that these new technologies fulfil no role. They certainly do, and should be developed and harnessed to help older people. But there is no way that they can take the place of ordinary human kindness and attention, and policy-makers and providers of care who believe that they can need to have a very serious rethink.

Quite how we can make better use of technology to give people more safety, choice and control at home, as well as making public spaces safe and accessible to older people, is not yet quite clear. The nightmare scenario would be to concentrate on the former – keeping old people safer at home, but in isolation – to such an extent that the issue about public spaces and making them safe and attractive to older people simply falls off the agenda. Then Roger Battersby's forecast will really come into being: older people will be safer in splendid isolation, and public space will only be for the young and fit. That is indeed a nightmare scenario.

Call to arms

The main question in all these areas – from toilets to telecare – is whether older people have managed to use their votes or their voices strongly enough to influence design for public space that meets their needs. A short look around the public realm makes it pretty clear that, for whatever reason, they haven't – certainly not in a proportion that reflects the size of the older population.

There may not be ageism endemic in the thinking about public spaces, though planning for the future tends to be couched in public debate in terms of the needs of children and young people. Nor are there fair and proper mechanisms to balance the different needs and priorities of different age groups in society in public space: often the potential conflicts are simply never discussed.

There is some hope from the Royal Town Planning Institute which wants Supplementary Planning Guidance for taking the ageing population into the planning system.[22] They want the development of specialist housing, both sheltered and otherwise, and 'lifetime neighbourhoods', so that housing and other facilities remain appropriate for people throughout their lifetimes, so people don't have to move neighbourhood as they age and can't manage their houses any longer.

But there is little evidence about the impact of regeneration schemes on public space for older people, where wholesale tearing down of old, sub-standard housing and public areas displaces older people who never totally recover from the move, although there are examples – such as the St Ann's Project in Nottingham in the 1960s – which show how this could and should be done. Nor is there much evidence yet that the growth of telecare isn't as much of a threat as an opportunity, despite the great praise which is lavished on it, by removing older people from public space.

There are not many real incentives for designers of all kinds to pay attention to the priorities of older people, particularly those who have a disability or sensory impairment. This is despite the sterling work of the Helen Hamlyn Foundation, the Disabled Living Foundation and others, all promoting the work of designers who do focus on such issues. Since the mid 1980s the Helen Hamlyn Foundation has spearheaded a campaign to make design fit the real lives of older people.[23] Along with the Conran Foundation, it ran the most splendid exhibition at the Victoria and Albert Museum as long ago as 1986 called 'Ten Million Characters in Search of a Design'. From kitchen fittings to knives for people with arthritis, from trainer-style shoes to gardening equipment to shower fittings, it was all there and well ahead of its time. Even so, a quick glance at the advertising in the pages of the National Trust magazine or the Sunday papers makes it clear that designing for people who are old and infirm does not bring out the best, or the most imaginative, in the design teams concerned.

That makes it all the more important that older people themselves influence design in all public spaces, and are loudly dissatisfied with anything less than the best. Older people need to take possession of these issues, and really make their voices heard. They need to insist that their needs are balanced against those of other groups, and that there is a real investigation into the impact of regeneration schemes on older people. They also need to get the charities that represent older people to provide incentives for designers to pay attention to what older people want, particularly anyone with a disability or a sensory impairment. Most of all, they are going to have to take those responsible for shops, town centres and shopping centres by the scruff of the neck and embarrass them into providing the facilities they need – toilets, chairs, a warm welcome and much more besides.

It is complete nonsense to suggest that younger people – however professional they are – can plan town centres or neighbourhoods with no advice from older people. But it is probably too much to expect them to realize that by themselves. Sophie Handler in Newham was absolutely right that older people need to reclaim the streets, if necessary by holding tea-dances in the local parks after dark. In fact, a range of ideas emerged from young people in the 1960s – like reclaiming the streets – that are, if anything, more relevant to older people now. Communal living may not be very attractive, after all, for younger people making their way in the world, but when you are older – and you need other people around who are mutually supportive – it may be very relevant indeed.

The manifesto also needs to find a better mechanism whereby older people can force their thinking on to the agenda at local authority level. **Every local council needs a standing committee of over-seventies, elected by local people who are over 70 themselves, which can compel any public official to answer questions and write an annual report on the state of the area from an older people's point of view.**

They should have the power to hold those who take the decisions to account, and to report on specific local issues like an American-style Grand Jury. This may not achieve their objectives directly or immediately, but it will give them considerable political and media power. Their annual reports should also go automatically to the Audit Commission.

Older people vote, and do so in greater numbers than younger people, yet something about local authorities makes them blind to this – able to close the public toilets, or leave older people marooned in the most horrific housing estates. The standing committee is designed to remind councils of their existence. The manifesto also needs to include demands to:

- **Force developers to show they have worked with local groups of older people before any planning application is given approval.** The resulting conversations may only result in tiny changes in the way new developments are built, but it is often very small changes that make a big difference to older people. Local authorities need to look at their own provision at the same time, and on the same basis – perhaps through the standing committees I suggested above – to see how they can improve basic things like toilets, park benches, benches on the street or flowerbeds in parks (raised flowerbeds can make a great deal of difference, for example). Are there seats in the bus stops? Do they have shelter? Are the paths in the parks designed only with skateboarders in mind? Involving older people may be all that is necessary to get these things right.

- **Insist on effective public transport in rural areas to suit older people.** This may just mean organizing bus timetables better or it may mean arranging for community transport to pick people up locally once a week and take them back again. It may be the kind of lift schemes that volunteers can and do organize for themselves. But it is local authorities that have the responsibility to make it happen, and they should be answerable to the standing committees for their record. Poor public transport in rural areas is often so bad that older people carry on driving far longer than they should for the safety of themselves and others. But what do we expect them to do? Stay at home?

- **Force local authorities to take responsibility for providing clean, safe, accessible public toilets.** Councils don't have to actually provide them themselves: they could pay or persuade local businesses to do it. If shops and other businesses are prevented from doing this because of insurance stipulations, as they sometimes claim, then the government needs to bring in the insurance companies and hammer out a deal to overcome this objection. Our miserable failure to provide public toilets now means we are trapping older people in their homes, at great cost to social and healthcare services. Yet we have summoned the political will to improve disabled access – why not toilets too?

- **Bring in older people to monitor and manage council services.** Our failure to do this so far means we are wasting the time and talents of older people, though you often find older people in rural areas – entirely on their own initiative – wandering round picking up litter with a pointed stick. Watford experimented with getting older people to monitor the performance of their rubbish collection services. We could definitely improve local parks by putting older people there to watch over them, in sufficient numbers to prevent them being cowed by groups of young people (though park-keeping is a paid job and they should be paid for it). All these roles need to be recognized and given status, and recompensed with something – whether it is parties or cheap entry into local sports centres or sports fixtures or credits through the local time bank. Older people treasure the places they live, so those places have to treasure them.

- **Insist on the accessibility of public transport.** It is completely indefensible that railway stations like Clapham Junction should be allowed to run with minimal toilet facilities and no way for anybody who isn't mobile to move from platform to platform.

- **Find new ways of encouraging older people to do T'ai Chi.** We know that T'ai Chi is very effective as a way of preventing older people having falls. We need to make it fun, and reward people for doing it regularly, offering them special sessions at museums, galleries and theatres.

Chapter 5

Don't make me brain dead, let me grow

Open access to learning

The best day of my life.

Winifred Warburton, 101, about the day she recorded 'My Generation' for the rock group The Zimmers at the famous Abbey Road studio in 2007

In the popular media a vision which pictures old people as a passive and pathological problem group characterized by dependency has been partially eclipsed by 'positive ageing' messages about the hedonistic joys of leisured retirement.

Andrew Blaikie, *Ageing and Popular Culture*, 1999

Buster Martin was born in France the year of the San Francisco earthquake in 1906, the year that the launch of the battleship *Dreadnought* began the naval arms race that ended with the First World War, and three years before the first British old age pensions. He came to London when he was three months old, had 17 children and now believes he is Britain's oldest employee – he works three days a week with Pimlico Plumbers, and refused to take the day off for his hundredth birthday.

In 2007, at the age of 101, he hit the headlines again as a member of the rock group The Zimmers, the brainchild of documentary maker Tim Samuels, which recorded their first hit single at the Abbey Road Studios and were an instant success. Their YouTube video has been downloaded 2 million times.

The Zimmers has 40 members with a combined age of more than 3,000 years (the lead singer is 90). As we go to press, they are still going strong, a testament that older people can do really anything. Living a good life when you are older is not just about telecare, or the provision of benches, seats and public toilets. A key part of what older people themselves say makes a difference, and keeps them healthy, is having a sense of purpose. Even the experts say that learning new things and 'mental excitement' are tremendously important.

But this is learning in the broadest sense. It means learning for the sake of it, not necessarily to make yourself employable, but so that you can play a wider role in society or be a more rounded person. It might be about learning skills as much as learning things: joining a choir, learning to sculpt or starting a rock group. It might be, like Peggy McAlpine, learning to paraglide off the coast of Cyprus a few days after her hundredth birthday.[1] It all keeps people active and healthy, builds society and asserts the idea of education as a lifelong activity.

This chapter is about learning when you are older, its importance, the possibilities and the barriers to spreading it more widely.

Informal learning

The University of the Third Age (U3A) is often described as a middle-class endeavour, but it has transformed thinking much more widely than those who are directly involved. The historian Peter Laslett coined the term 'Third Age' to define the time for personal fulfilment before the onset of the degenerative Fourth Age. He founded the institution in 1981, together with Michael Young and Eric Midwinter, based on the idea that older people have sufficient health, wealth and time to determine new lifestyles in such a way as to achieve personal fulfilment.

Actually, of course, U3A includes people who are well into what you might call the Fourth Age as well. Its importance is that it rests on a vision of older people as having the opportunities, and an awareness of them, and the ability to make all sorts of choices. The tragedy is that this vision is not shared everywhere, and especially not for many people living in deprived areas. The researchers Botham and Lumley, whom I have quoted elsewhere, draw the conclusion:

> *It may be said, therefore, that the third age is a phenomenon only for certain sections of the population, sections that do not include the most deprived, isolated and excluded. For these people, ageing is more likely to involve an accelerated transition from the second towards the fourth age.*[2]

The challenge is therefore to extend this vision of the possibility of learning, and other personal fulfilment opportunities, to older people for whom they are not now a reality. Age Concern has tried to do more to help people who want to do more learning, even if they are disabled or financially deprived. Their 'Leisure and Learning' fact sheet is full of information on doing further courses and study, from formal to informal, from getting a grant for studying to learning about heritage days, from exploring family history on the web to taking part in sport or literary events. Though not everyone finds it easy, the evidence is clear that there is a growing number of older people who want to learn more, study more, and engage either in serious scholarship or in more informal research about their own backgrounds, neighbourhood or the area of the country from where their family came originally. Yet there are real issues about the availability of courses and help and advice for such projects, and the government has been shifting educational funding from older to younger people. This is an area where older people's charities really should have been making a huge fuss, given all the evidence about active minds slowing down mental degeneration, and given the human cost of older people's isolation and boredom.

Various voluntary organizations are doing a great deal to make that personal fulfilment a reality for some of those in more deprived and isolated areas. The Sundial Centre in Bethnal Green in east London, for example, has won considerable praise from government ministers for the diversity of services it provides and for going out and becoming part of the wider community. 'The Sundial Singers are giving a soaring, emotion-filled rendition of "The Water is Wide", a traditional Irish song about lost love,' wrote Mark Gould in the *Guardian* after a visit there in 2006.[3] 'Nearby, the three sisters of the knitting circle – June White, Vera Caley and Vi Davis – are busy knitting clothes. There is a queue for hairdresser Martha, who is offering a shampoo and set for £8.50, and the keep-fit class is a wind farm of whirling arms. There are wholesome smells coming from the cafeteria, where lunch is being prepared.'

The Sundial was set up in 2001 as a partnership between the Peabody Trust, Tower Hamlets council social services and London Catalyst, previously known as the Metropolitan Hospitals Sunday Fund. It offers 30 social service day-centre places, but can accommodate more than 100 people for big events or open days, and professional referrals to day activities are not required. The centre's computer classes are available to everyone over 25. There is also a self-help group for arthritis, a hearing aid clinic, aromatherapy, T'ai Chi, and a community newspaper written by and for Sundial users.

But where it fits well into the Third Age self-fulfilment model, even for deprived older people, is that some of its users have passed GCSEs in citizenship as a result of work with nearby Oaklands secondary school. Pupils from the school also come into the Sundial to learn about the lives of people who have lived through world wars, unemployment and strife. And those not in the least deprived make use of similar facilities, such as Pilates classes in nearby community centres.

Pilates, incidentally, was all the rage amongst the well-heeled some ten years ago, but it has real attractions for older people because it doesn't involve bouncing up and down aerobic exercises which can be difficult as joints get stiffer. In fact, the government might usefully add Pilates to the list of services available on the NHS.

The point is that learning does not have to be the conventional kind. It can mean anything that broadens people, stretches their mind or gives them skills. Not only will this keep them healthy, but it will also bring them into contact with local organizations – even schools – to their mutual benefit.

Libraries

The conventional picture is of older people, frail and lonely, using the public library to keep warm. Some elements of this are still around. Certainly, a large number of older people use public libraries to read the newspapers, as they always have done. Getting hard data on this was far from easy, but the National Statistics publication *Focus on Older People* said that there were 149 million visits to libraries in 2004 by people over 55, and around 30 per cent of library users were over the age of 65.[4]

They are such an important clientele for libraries that the Chartered Institute of Librarians and Information Professionals has set out guidelines for their members on how older people use libraries, and should be encouraged to use them.[5] This includes such fairly obvious guidance as avoiding stereotyping. But it also argues that 'the information needs of older people have traditionally been seen as relating to information about benefits, pensions or care. These are important for some, but older people are not a homogenous group – for many retirement is a time of great opportunity.'

Quite so. But the importance of libraries to older people sometimes eludes policy-makers who don't happen to be librarians themselves. The report on the two-year action research programme known as Better Government for Older People – Warwick University's publication called *Making a Difference* (2000) – listed all 28 of the local pilots, but there was almost no link with library services.[6] When Rebecca Linley wrote about older people, libraries and social exclusion that same year, she was clearly right that all those cross-cutting council initiatives on lifelong learning, safety, independent living and supporting people needed to link better with libraries.[7]

She also urged libraries to make sure that any English language published material uses 14pt or 16pt and a sanserif typeface, so that one print version is accessible to as many people as possible. Most older people should be able to use libraries with no more help than the average person, with good guiding, a subject index and an inquiry desk, she said. But they might want a higher proportion of leisure or information materials:

> *Some learn new skills which they never had time for*
> *before – they might study for an Open University degree,*
> *write books – Mary Wesley started writing in her 70s – or*
> *read all the works of Dickens. Some are in fact busier*
> *than ever with family commitments or voluntary work.*
> *Some may need particular formats – spoken word, large*
> *print books, coffee table or illustrated books.*[8]

But many libraries are rising to this challenge. Essex has two 'silver surfer' clubs. Rhondda Cynon Taff's IT classes for older people, in partnership with Age Concern, began in one library and were so popular that they were extended to other branches. Hampshire has two reading groups run specifically for visually impaired people, and Warwickshire has reading chains and groups for older people in the community, including housebound people. West Sussex has a housebound readers group, in partnership with a local voluntary organization, which provides adult education to housebound people. The organization uses its own transport to take a group of readers to their own premises once a month – the library service provides the books and a member of staff to lead the group.

Many older people are engaged in research. But libraries may need equipment such as magnifiers and enlarging photocopiers and induction loops, seating at a variety of heights, some with arm rests, some without, and more trolleys or baskets for carrying chosen books. In fact, Kent provides trolleys based on the Zimmer frame principle with a high-slung basket, which is particularly useful in larger libraries where people have to walk some distance.

But why not go further? There is no reason why libraries should not provide refreshments and, as I outlined in the last chapter, the failure to provide toilets is a real deterrent for older people. Even in the United States, with its general lack of public provision, most libraries manage to have public toilet facilities. Why not here?

There is also far too little emphasis on mobile and home library services, which can make an enormous difference to people's lives. As evidence of this, one answer received from a user survey by the Westminster Home Library Service said this:

> *The service has been one of the great comforts of my life.*
> *I have always been a lover of reading and to know that*
> *every three weeks a stack of books of my choice are being*
> *delivered to me I am certain helps me to enjoy life in*
> *spite of the usual sorrow and disabilities of old age.*

Alan Bennett's highly successful short novella about the Queen and the mobile library may seem fanciful to some, but its serious point about the easy availability of books is important. Mobile libraries make such a difference to older people of all social groups, and they need to be available in towns and cities as well as in rural areas, to give older people the chance to read, change their books, and talk to librarians – who are also a vastly underappreciated source of mental stimulation and friendship for older people. Indeed, as my parents grew old, the librarians at the library at the end of their street in London used to hand deliver books to them, because they were so concerned that they could no longer get out.

Libraries are not alone. Many museums and galleries have major programmes of informal learning which attract older people. Some are free and some are very low cost, but many of these institutions see it as part of their mission to run programmes like that – again, something that government is unclear about in cost terms, because it is increasingly choosing not to subsidize them. Amongst the best examples of this are the programmes run at the Dulwich Picture Gallery, a major collection, yet not one of our national museums. From art appreciation discussion groups for retired people to master classes and 'painting for the petrified', they draw in people of all kinds and all ages, including large numbers of older people, believing that people who are in danger of losing their self-esteem can change their view of themselves if they hang them, metaphorically speaking – according to the *Daily Telegraph* – among the Rembrandts and Poussins.

Working with Dulwich Homelink, a befriending organization for housebound older people, they brought housebound people into the gallery. The Imperial War Museum, the V&A, the National Gallery, the Tate and many of the museums up and down the country do the same. This is a godsend for opening older people's eyes, but – given the government's priorities for education for employability – it is now under threat.

Formal learning

There was a fascinating media tussle in 2006 after the *Daily Telegraph* declared that the former High Court judge Sir Oliver Popplewell, 78, currently an undergraduate at Harris Manchester College in Oxford, studying politics, philosophy and economics, was the oldest student at Oxford University. The report was followed shortly afterwards by a letter from Professor Michael Vickers, of

Jesus College. 'I am the supervisor of Miss Gertrud Seidmann of Wolfson College,' he wrote, 'who is studying for a [higher degree] at the age of 86.'

Gertrud Seidmann has been pursuing an MLitt, which will probably become a DPhil, on the life and achievements of Greville Chester, a nineteenth-century clergyman 'who became an assiduous traveller to Egypt and the near east, and an expert on archaeological artefacts which he collected for museums'. She spends her days working at her home in the city, or at the university's libraries, and attending public lectures in the Ashmolean Museum and Oxford's various colleges.

'I came here to teach in the first place,' she says, 'but the attraction of Oxford is obvious: contact with the best scholars, combined with college life and its stimulating company of men and women of quite varying professional and private interests.'

A retired schoolteacher and an academic, she changed course to study engraved gems and eighteenth-century collectors. Rather deaf as she got older, she is finding that technology can overcome her loss of hearing, which makes telephone conversations difficult, and allowed for her interview with me to be conducted via what she called 'the blessed email'. She does not often meet with the bulk of the university's 11,119 undergraduate students, but sometimes with much younger postgraduates:

> At my stage in life, I prefer my own house and garden.
> But I go into college almost every day. Lunch with an
> ever-varying, entertaining company in hall – and the food
> is very good! – use the library and common rooms, and
> walk in the beautiful grounds. I continue to do what I
> have been doing for the previous 25 years – research,
> write and lecture. As I have been a fellow of the Society of

Antiquaries and an honorary research associate of the university Institute of Archaeology for many years, my life has not really changed all that much. There is just the added bonus of detailed attention to, and criticism of, my work.

But one thing has changed: her tutors appear a little younger than they once were. 'Of course I am older than my supervisor, who will have to retire at 67 or so,' she says. 'Poor man.'

Gertrud Seidmann, who very generously agreed to be interviewed for this book, felt she also needed to be clear that there was a little bit of the downside. She has lived alone for decades, with a few exceptions, which is 'not all that great all the time, for practical reasons', though she clearly enjoys her own company, and has friends and colleagues with whom to discuss everything under the sun. Relatives are few and far between, none close, scattered around the globe, and friends are dying off, though she has close younger friends. Nor is she free of depression, particularly in the summer, and is not very domesticated. But mostly she is upbeat about making constant discoveries and in regular contact with interesting old and new acquaintances. She is about to finalize a catalogue of the Soane Museum gems with Martin Henig. She also writes prolifically about her beloved Chester and others, with a fierceness and clarity younger people should envy.[9]

Despite being seen and publicized as somewhat extraordinary for pursuing her degree – which she is doing because she is interested in the subject and wants to publish more on it – Gertrud Seidmann is really doing what she has done all her life. She does not want to be famous for fifteen minutes for being old, like many of the other older people who I spoke to for this book. It is an accolade for Oxford in general, and Wolfson College in particular, that they think there is nothing odd in an 86 year old doing a master's degree, but perhaps they should encourage more people, active intellectually and with scholarly interests, to do just the same.

Researching for this book turned up huge numbers of older people doing just that. The advice so often given to younger people to do Sudoku puzzles to keep the brain active is as nothing compared to the large numbers of older people – some of whom are really very old indeed, even by modern standards – writing, researching, taking degrees, arguing, debating and generally having a thoroughly satisfactory and even exciting intellectual life.

The higher education figures show that in 2004/5 there were 27,320 undergraduate students over 61, and another 2,975 postgraduate students over the same age. There is also a smallish number whose ages are unknown: about 10,000 in total. So, although the percentage of older people studying at conventional universities is relatively small, it is by no means negligible – those who want to do it and can afford it are able to carry on with their formal education beyond any normal retirement age.

The overall numbers in formal education have grown hugely. There are now officially more than 600,000 learners over the age of 60 in England alone.[10] Often these are people who are going to college for the first time, or finally studying what they always wanted to do when parental pressure pushed them in another direction. Like Rosemary Mackinder, 61, who worked as a civil servant because her father thought being an artist was not a proper job. But having retired, she took an access course in art at Colchester Institute, and was one of only two students in her year to pass with distinction. She has now begun a three-year degree course. 'I loved mixing with the younger students. It was so involving for me, and I think that worked both ways.' The Open University now takes three per cent of its students from the over-65s and six per cent from the 55–64 age group.

This is an inspiring picture, but the trend is not necessarily going in the right direction. The government has decided to refocus its attention on younger learners, and funding cuts have been looming in colleges and further education. It was already clear, just from the figures for 2004–6, that the number of people over 25 pursuing adult and further education courses had dropped by nearly a million because of fee increases and government policies to concentrate public funds on a few priorities.

The Department for Education and Skills was celebrating the increases in the numbers of students doing longer high-priority courses 'in line with the government's funding priorities to drive up the nation's productivity and global competitiveness', and ignored this overall decline. But Alan Tuckett, director of NIACE (the National Institute of Adult Continuing Education) said this was too high a price to pay. He warned that all the gains of the previous ten years were being lost, apart from improvements in literacy, language and numeracy, and said that adult learning provision had been devastated over the previous two years.[11]

Worse, the numbers of over-50s attending evening classes has dropped by a third over the last two years, mainly because of the increases in fees charged for these courses – the so-called 'non-priority courses' – and the closure of colleges fearful of failing to attract enough of the right kind of high-priority students. Alan Tuckett asked whether these policies were sensible, given that 'we can all expect a further 30 years of life beyond retirement'.

He was right to ask, because the government has been making it increasingly clear that their main objective is to 'promote economically valuable skills'.[12] All this simply ignores the facts: older people can both be economically valuable in the workplace and as mentors for younger people, not to mention the great economic saving of keeping them mentally active and alert so that they do not cost the public purse money in terms of health and social care. Of all the short-sighted decisions examined in this volume, this one may well turn out to be the most stupid, and the least holistic.

Dance

Older people sail, canoe, climb mountains, lift weights, play tennis, and are generally very active. The image of the old lady sitting in her chair, quietly dozing over her knitting, is a long way from the truth. An Irish friend of ours in her seventies spent many happy hours showing me how to melt sulphur in a spade over a naked flame to kill off bees stuck up my chimney, and seemed not at all phased by the fact that many people 30 years her junior would find that hard, taxing and dangerous work.

There is also a positive revival of interest in dance amongst older people. Or, perhaps, more accurately, a desire to dance and not enough facilities for doing so. The Arts Council has shown that dance activity can adapt to the abilities and needs of older people, and that increasing activity levels both help to reduce the risk of fractures due to falls and reduce isolation and build confidence and self-esteem. The Attik Dance Company delivered weekly dance classes for older people in Plymouth throughout 2003 and 2004, targeting deprived areas or areas where there was a lack of activity for older people, a fairly constant complaint. Class tutors built up a 'library' of movement to develop people's key skills, before gradually introducing them to more creative activity. Participants felt that their overall fitness and energy levels had improved, and also that the classes had partly alleviated their health problems. They also helped them to create new, sustainable social relationships.

Meanwhile, Dr Helen Thomas and other academics at Goldsmiths College in London looked at dance more generally and how older people take up what is on offer.[13] They showed that plenty of over-60s were travelling across London and Essex in buses, trains, underground and cars, sometimes three or four times a week, to take part in their favourite dance events. Their mapping exercise revealed just how much the over-60s are involved in social dance as an activity that was previously invisible, culturally and academically.

A dance company called From Here to Maturity was formed in 2000 to provide opportunities for older dancers. It deliberately challenges ageism and prejudice by designing original and imaginative dance pieces, as well as through both education and outreach. The company's outstanding dancers range in age between the late forties and early seventies, and include former principals, soloists and stars of the Royal Ballet and Ballet Rambert.

So popular has dance become for older people that NIACE commissioned some research into it, and the response was huge. People made it very clear that dancing was not only an Olympic event, but also recognized as an aerobic activity. Others particularly replied that salsa dancing was something you could do without a partner, and that it is supportive, as is tap dancing, and – when most class members were female – they wanted to have an activity where the absence of a partner isn't an issue. This was another benefit cited for Circle Dancing, done in most towns but not well known. There was also a great deal about the benefits of flexibility and mobility, as well as better stamina, making friends, lifting the spirits and improving brain power.

'Remember, dancing isn't only done on and with the feet,' said another. 'You should see my seated can-can!'

It is hardly surprising, given this enthusiasm, that the Scottish parliament has been receiving petitions calling for a National Dance

Hall. One of the organizers, Joyce Kinnear, explained that the normal venues have yet to realize the economic potential:

> We suggest that nightclub owners have yet to see the
> potential financial benefits of providing activity for this
> large section of the population, who have disposable
> income and plenty of time and energy to dispose of it.
> The view amongst venue owners appears to be that older
> people are unwilling to come out and that such a night
> would not provide high bar takings. This is a self-fulfilling
> prophecy, as older people don't go out to nightclubs
> because the music and environment is not set up to fulfil
> their needs.[14]

I had not expected to read so much on dance for older people when researching for this book. It is extraordinarily heart-warming to read just how much is going on, and the fact that people are dancing even if considerably disabled, in residential and care homes, and in wheelchairs. This surely adds weight to older people's own views that it is the quality of life that must be addressed, and physical activity is a key part of that.

Internet and computer games

One of the strangest phenomena of recent years is the over-45s getting hooked on computer games. This is a particularly Japanese trend, moving into Europe and the USA, fuelled by the idea that if you take up 'brain training' you will ward off the effects of old age. Nintendo has designed and marketed a package of cerebral workouts which is said to improve mental agility and even to slow the onset and progress of Alzheimer's disease and dementia more widely. Players have to complete puzzles as quickly and accurately as possible, including reading literary classics aloud, doing simple arithmetic, drawing and responding rapidly to deceptively easy teasers using voice-recognition software. The games then decide the player's 'brain age'.

What is obviously so addictive is that a physically-fit cerebrally challenged 30 year old might be told after his first few attempts that his brain is into his fifties, while a retired woman, with a bit of practice, could end up with a brain age 20 years younger than she actually is. Which was partly what the inventor intended: he is a 46-year-old professor of neuroscience at Tohoku University, who had spent years looking at the benefits of solving straightforward mathematical and other problems.[15] Some commentators have been a bit sceptical, even in Japan, saying that this is about denial. But there is evidence that keeping the brain active may well help delay the onset of dementia if it is coming, quite apart from being fun itself.

Older people using the internet is another major change, and may be one of the transformational drivers in changing life for older people more generally. One survey suggests that 41 per cent of retired British people say that surfing the internet is amongst their favourite pastimes.[16] Gardening and DIY have slipped to 39 per cent. In fact, it was a decade ago that Microsoft discovered that the over-60s were spending more time at their computers than any other age group: ten hours a week, compared with the then average of seven hours. eBay found that a third of British pensioners were willing to sell their possessions on their site to pay for holidays and other treats.

Older people are making dates online, broadcasting online and webcasting. In fact, the internet is heaving with older people, and may be a sign of what is in store for other aspects of life. It is a technology that is designed for people who may not always be able to go out, and it empowers them to do all sorts of research and be far more demanding than they might have been in a previous life.

Outward bound

In February 2006, Shealagh Ward, 68, and her husband Alan, 64, were left stranded in the Atlantic Ocean in their catamaran without power, steering, or fresh water, after setting out on a trip around the world.[17] The couple had retired four years before after running pubs across the UK, and had set off from Cape Verde bound for Trinidad and Tobago. Their adventure came to an abrupt end seven days into their journey across the Atlantic when their boat lost propulsion and steering.

They were rescued by the merchant ship *Castillo de San Pedro*, which was diverted by coastguards to their last known position. 'That was their dream, to sail around the world,' their son Stuart told the media. 'At the end of the day, knowing them, it's not something they would have done lightly but also, knowing them and how safety conscious they are, and how they both prepared, I was very concerned. But by the same token, if anyone was going to make it, they would.'

Despite an appalling ordeal, their son thought they would simply recover and try again. Time and again, there are accounts of older people having a dream of doing something, and trying again and again to achieve it. Mountains, lakes, oceans – all of them are challenges for a whole new generation of older people who do not see their later years as any reason to stop being active. Indeed, for many older people, retirement has given them the opportunity to be more active, fitter, happier and taking on greater and greater challenges.

But there is a problem. Older travellers wanting to do exciting things have a real problem with insurance. About 70 per cent of single-trip insurance policies impose an upper age limit, and 90 per cent of the more economical, annual multi-trip policies also impose upper age limits. Help the Aged found that one in four annual policies will not cover the over-65s while about 70 per cent will not cover the over-75s.

We are an ageing society. Seventy is supposed to be the new fifty. Yet many older people are being discouraged from being adventurous and going to distant places or doing mildly dangerous sports because they can't get insurance, or because it is so expensive that it discourages them, and they don't feel it is fair to their nearest and dearest to take trips abroad without basic insurance cover that would deal with hospital costs and repatriation if necessary.

There are a few providers which do provide annual cover, though it is expensive, particularly if it includes the United States, because healthcare costs are so high there. Saga is one key provider; Age Concern and Help the Aged are both using their trading arms to fill this gap. But the scandal is that people are being charged large sums, even though they are generally no less fit than 50 or 60 year olds were a generation ago, who faced no such discrimination.

Being unfit and isolated

'During your morning ablutions, you think of several things you need to do today and by the time you're finished at the wash basin they have gone,' wrote Blake Morrison, reviewing a series of books about old age.[18] 'You console yourself that Titian was painting at 88, Adenauer running Germany at 87, Alistair Cooke broadcasting weekly at 95, John Gielgud still acting a month before he died at 96.'

These are the wealthy, successful role models, alongside Churchill who painted and drank till the end, and others who write, pray, talk, argue, read, go to exhibitions and concerts and whatever. The problem is that it isn't all like that, and some of it depends on money. If you have far less money, what is an active and good old age like? And how do we try to do better for the less affluent, given the appalling statistic that the poorest ten per cent are more than twice as likely to die before the age of 65 than the richest ten per cent?

The other side of the coin is that at least 2 million older people in the UK are so isolated that they only see anyone – family, friends or neighbours – once a week or less. Old age can also deepen exclusion from the normal support structures, and make poverty and isolation even worse. Older women, the over-75s, older people with disabilities, those from black and minority ethnic backgrounds and some other groups are more likely to be trapped in this vicious cycle.

Worse, those charitable organizations which are trying to do something about it in deprived areas, or in pockets of deprivation, find it really difficult to raise the money, because older people are not popular as a charitable cause. Phrases like 'the elderly' or 'the aged' are deliberately distancing; those people are not like you and me.

The WRVS, leaders in provision of meals on wheels and other services for isolated older people, has challenged public, private and not-for-profit service providers to make sure that all older people in the UK have daily human contact by 2010.[19] If 32 older people in the UK die alone and unnoticed in their homes every day – the equivalent of 12,000 a year – as they say, then that is a very serious condemnation of the way we organize society for older people. Ten per cent of those responding to the NOP survey on the subject said that their WRVS volunteer was the person they saw most often during the week.

The key difference between active and lonely older people is their mobility and whether they can get out of the house. While 63 per cent of the general public spend less than half of a typical day in their home, three quarters of WRVS's customers rarely or never leave their home. 'Few understand the multiple impacts that loneliness can have, it can be the difference between life and death,' said WRVS's then chief executive Mark Lever:

> Housebound and deprived of human contact, older
> people go downhill rapidly in both physical and mental
> terms, and can quite literally lose the will to live.
> Loneliness amongst older people is accompanied by a
> loss of confidence and we know that over one in ten
> people over 65 suffers from depression ... It is up to all of
> us to consider how the needs of older people can be met
> through increased personal contact, giving them the
> choice to live independently and with dignity. No matter
> who you are, a visit to older family members or
> neighbours can make a real difference.[20]

But this requires more people, professionals and volunteers, formal and informal volunteers, to do more. If we want a more inclusive, more supportive society for older people, particularly those who are housebound or deprived in other ways, we need to get wider society to take this seriously. The WRVS asked, in that same NOP poll, how the general public would feel if they were as isolated as so many older people are. If they had to spend just a week in their house without visitors or being able to go out, 53 per cent said they would be really bored, 47 per cent said they would be lonely, and 20 per cent said they would get claustrophobic. Why should older people be any different?

As the WRVS hinted, isolation can become so bad that you can die without being noticed. Gerald Noble lay dead in his flat for five months before anyone knew about it.[21] With no traceable relatives, his funeral was left to the local authority to organize. He had been happier alone than in company, but had been a regular at the working men's club in his town of Rochdale, or in the pub on the estate where he lived. 'I noticed he didn't come in and out so much,' said one neighbour, a man of about the same age. 'But I just thought he had gone away.'

Nor was his fate that unusual. Nearly 200 councils responded to Sutton MP Paul Burstow when he asked how many funerals they had carried out for people who had no family or friends, and more than 11,000 such funerals had taken place over a five-year period, some 43 a week. The majority were for older men, who were two and a half times more likely to die alone than women.

Since more of us are living alone much earlier in life, this loneliness can be expected to increase in old age. More than a million Scots are expected to live on their own within two decades, according to the latest statistics, and over-60s will make up much of the overwhelming increase. The change is largely due to the fact that people are living longer and staying in their own homes into their old age, but many people are also marrying later or choosing to stay single.

But it is worse than that. The isolation is deeper because neighbourhoods are not as close-knit as they used to be, according to Alan Findlay, from the Centre for Applied Population Research at Dundee University.[22] 'Society undoubtedly faces a challenge as it adapts to more people living on their own in the latter part of their life,' he said. 'At a time when society is more individualistic at all ages, that does mean people are not as bound into a community. Older people do not necessarily know their neighbours or the younger members of their communities due to the high level of mobility that exists. That is an issue and a problem society as a whole faces.'

One way of coping for many, if they can manage the care, is to have a pet. The Cinnamon Trust helps old people care for their pets, organizing volunteers to dog walk for a housebound owner, take pets in when their owners need hospital care, fetching the cat food, cleaning out the bird cages or taking the pets to the vet. When old people have to go into a nursing or care home, Cinnamon provides a list of pet-friendly registered care and nursing homes, and also pet sanctuaries when things get too tough for the pets to stay with their owners, or the owner dies.

This is such an obvious way of dealing with some of the worst loneliness that it is amazing that it isn't better known. With 8,000 volunteers, the Cinnamon Trust could not possibly do all the caring for pets that might be needed, but it certainly does something original that gives great pleasure – and tackles the very worst features of being alone and housebound.

It is hardly surprising that, for the better off, there is a commercial opportunity in all this. The American company Home Instead Senior Care is now expanding in Australia, providing paid companions to lonely old people.[23] Beyond the usual homecare tasks of cooking, cleaning and laundry, the biggest need is for carers who will play Scrabble with their client, take them to the races, walk in the park with them and talk about old times.

This kind of service may seem like a godsend to overworked baby boomers who are earning too much to take their dad to the races or to play Scrabble with their mum, or who live too far away to visit regularly. They can pay someone else to keep loneliness at bay and social connection alive for their ageing parents. But it represents another shifting of the outsourcing boundary, and it begs the question of how far is too far in the commercialization of intimate life.

'A "paid" friend is an oxymoron,' wrote Adele Horin in the *Sydney Morning Herald*. 'A personal relationship built on commerce must always be suspected of being phoney at heart.'

The paid companion might actually build a genuine friendship with the person they are caring for – that often happened in previous generations of Victorian paid companions. They might prove to be more attentive, more involved and more valued than the absent son or daughter. It might work, but from a policy point of view it isn't an answer. How did the person get so isolated in the first place? And what can we do if we can't afford paid companions for everybody who is lonely? It seems extraordinary that older people should be expected to use their scarce resources to pay people to keep them company when volunteers, neighbours or others engaged through time banks and similar mutual support organizations are not just free, but probably more effective.

Intergenerational activities

The solution, once again, is in mobilizing very much larger numbers of volunteers than we have managed to do so far, many of them older people themselves. It is also in linking up the generations again, and here there is some hope. I was at a meeting of the all-party group on social exclusion amongst older people in 2006 listening to some of what was going on, and it sounded magnificent. Sheila Gent spoke about the intergenerational projects delivered by Age Concern Kingston since their inception in 1999. This work included a school-based project that was delivered initially through the Mount Primary School. The aim is to put teams of older volunteers into schools to support children from their first year through to year 6, giving reading support, help in science and technology, literacy and numeracy lessons plus, of course, pastoral support.

Age Concern Kingston rejoices in the fact that they buck a trend. Research suggests that many more women than men are likely to volunteer for such work, yet in Kingston they managed a good gender balance, with the numbers of volunteers steadily increasing. This was all so successful that, in 2005, they began to plan for the extension of their Age and Youth school-based project to include a Learning Mentor Project. Seven mentors began work with 13 children from the Mount Primary School, agreeing to carry on supporting them beyond primary school into the first year of their secondary education. This was felt to be an important bridge for the children at what was often a difficult transition period.

There are plenty of other examples of intergenerational practice, including craft partnerships, in which older people share their craft skills such as knitting, sewing and crocheting with younger people – practical engagement helps to bridge the gaps between generations and is much enjoyed by both age groups. There are also intergenerational discussion forums, which encourage younger and older people to come together. These provide an opportunity for younger and older people to talk about important, potentially conflicting viewpoints in a relaxed and friendly environment.

One of the great experiments is inter-generational learning, piloted in the International Baccalaureate schools. They recruited older people as tutors, companions, teachers, running orientation programmes, giving professional counselling and training in ethnic awareness. Pupils were also active in return, visiting community facilities, including hospitals and nursing homes, visiting older people, acting as companions, acting as tutors, helping older people learn new skills, such as computer skills, which are very popular, and collaborating in community service projects. There has also been a series of inter-generational conferences.

By far the most popular responses were for the combination of music, drama and sport, and these are programmes prepared by the students for the older people, usually, but not only, grandparents and great-grandparents. The evaluation suggests an increase in students' poise and self-respect. 'We have seen in practice what the theorists have been saying, that the intergenerational activities are a benefit to everyone,' said the report.[24] 'The interaction has enhanced the school's reputation, the students' self-confidence, and the seniors' appreciation of young people, as well as their technological skills.' It is fascinating how much this activity comes back, once again, to learning.

Arts projects, such as the London based 'Magic-Me', offer the opportunity to challenge social perceptions of the young and old, and this is important for building strength and respect in communities. There are support projects where older people support young mothers aged 13 and 14, or vulnerable younger people leaving local authority care. Then there is the Newport Equal Project where older volunteers share their skills with recent immigrants (especially bike repair, which gives them vital local skills). Or Sixty Plus, in Kensington and Chelsea, focusing on reading support, language development, IT support and art, which linked up with a crime diversion project to bag and deliver garden mulch to older people. Younger people taking part afterwards said they had learned a great deal about the less salubrious things the older participants had done in their youth.

Alan Hatton-Yeo, director of the Beth Johnson Foundation, talks about the importance of inter-generational projects for bridging the gap between generations – and calming the potential conflicts between them for scarce resources – and building a sense of shared history, especially locally. Older people taking part have been shown to get significant mental and physical health benefits. It also cuts down social isolation. He singled out the inter-generational book groups which took place in residential homes for older people, in which younger people and older people came together to discuss their experiences of reading a book each month.

It is a vital exchange that is going on: both older and younger people have something, potentially, that their opposite numbers need. What is lacking is often the funding to bring the two sides together.

Call to arms

There is a very great deal going on, and some of it very simple – like having older people joining schoolchildren for their school dinners, as in one Herefordshire village, which both the older people and the children seem to love. This is not an area where there is no hope, and it is clear that both young and old gain hugely from projects like this. The complaints were almost entirely about a lack of funding to organize this work, and one thing that is clear from everything I read for this volume is that the shortage of money for the things that make life 'feel better' is the most worrying of all.

Everyone accepts that money is needed for healthcare, for heating, for housing – though by no means enough – and for food. But the money, often quite small amounts, that makes life more fun, that encourage inter-generational mixing to everyone's advantage, that turns eating from simply swallowing necessary fuel into a social activity, seems in particularly short supply.

Those who have money find it easier, but even they benefit from this kind of mentoring or inter-generational projects where the organization has to be carefully managed and people have to be supported and trained. The less well off are the most likely to be socially excluded, and for them the money to make these projects possible seems absolutely essential.

Inter-generational projects are as much about learning as the University of the Third Age or colleges, but it is more formal learning in colleges which is currently under threat from a narrow view of what education is, and a blinkered idea of the disposability of older people. That is the only explanation for the shift in government policy which is making local colleges and further education much more narrowly focused on slotting young people into employment.

This is not to suggest that educating young people for the employment market isn't important. Of course it is. But there are other purposes to education in a civilized and healthy society, where people are in education – in one way or another – for most of their lives. Young people need more than just skills for employers, and older people need the same fuel for the human spirit which is being squeezed out of further education by deliberate policy. Most of the central government funding is now going towards employment-related courses, so that if you want to do book-binding or printing or music you are perceived by the government, quite wrongly, as selfishly pursuing it for yourself alone, and you will have to pay the full costs.

Some will do that, where those life-enhancing courses remain – and they are being squeezed out everywhere – but many will not, and many older people won't ask for a subsidy even if one is available, and usually it isn't. This completely cuts across the idea at the heart of this book, that everyone – definitely including older people – will be healthier, happier and more effective (and less costly to the state) when they are active, inspired and learning. That is especially so if society is going to persuade people to stay in paid employment for longer.

So a key plank in this manifesto is that **older people should be able to access a wide range of education and learning at a** reasonable cost, and to learn whatever it is that inspires them to grow as people – not just what the Department for Education happens to approve of as 'useful' from one moment to the next. Of course, it is also reasonable that they should have to pay, but it is counter-productive to expect older people on pensions to pay the full costs. Such a policy is more humane, more life-affirming, and also in the long-run a good deal healthier – and therefore cheaper to the public purse – than a narrowing of education to its most youthful and utilitarian.

The manifesto should also include demands to:

- **Launch systems that allow volunteers to earn credits for their efforts which can be used to access further education.** Time banks already recognize people's efforts with credits that they can use to access volunteer help themselves when they need it, but this needs to be extended to colleges – as in some parts of the United States – so that people can use those credits to take part in courses. This will reward volunteers, encourage more to feel they are recognized, and encourage older people to learn.

- **End discrimination against older people in travel insurance.** There is no excuse for denying people travel insurance just on the basis of their age, rather than their actual state of health. The current policy is lazy and discriminatory, and is undermining the efforts to keep older people active. Once again, the government needs to bring the insurance companies together and hammer out some kind of solution.

- **Carry out serious cost-benefit analyses of inter-generational projects.** One of the reasons these are difficult to fund, at least sustainably, is that policy-makers in central and national government are unaware of the wider economic effects they have, in reducing crime, improving education and prolonging health in old age. It is time we knew that for certain, so that government could invest serious money in such schemes, and make sure there is – at the very least – an inter-generational project attached to every primary and secondary school, public and private.

- **Extend the role of neighbourhood watch.** It may not be learning in the narrow sense, but there is a wider role for organizations like Neighbourhood Watch to seek out older people who are isolated and get them involved in activities or learning, linking with Age Concern, WRVS or local time banks.

Chapter 6

Don't force me into a care home

Real choice in housing

Eighteen months ago, I was completely bedridden, stuck between four walls, and I became invisible. I suddenly became terribly aware of what it was like to be old and isolated and have a total lack of stimulation.

Clare Du Boulay, a member of the experimental Vivariaum housing group, *Glasgow Herald*, 23 June 2004

In this country, as women get older they outlive men and tend to end up living by themselves. I don't want to end up with my kids looking after me, and me still being lonely. I would like my friends to be there in future, if I can arrange it like that. This is a way of doing that. I'll have my own front door but my mates will be on tap.

Jane Nelson, member of the London co-housing group OWCH, *Observer*, 20 May 2004

When I was still a student, I was involved as a volunteer in the St Ann's project in Nottingham, an enormous redevelopment scheme which moved people out of the area before the rebuilding and moved them back in afterwards. I helped pack up the homes of some of the older people who lived there, and helped move them back again after their homes had been renovated. Even now, I can remember the sheer joy they felt about going home – the idea that they could carry on living in their home neighbourhood as they got older, and that the familiar people would be around them too.

It is said that people become more wedded to their possessions as they get older. I don't think that's quite accurate, but home certainly does become more important. Why did my father feel unable to die until he had come home? Because people need to feel they are where they belong. Yet in so many cases we expect older people to move out completely, into distant sheltered accommodation or 'retirement villages' where little is familiar, and then – because the basic care isn't available – to uproot themselves again into a care home.

It is deeply traumatic, corrosive of people's health and undermining of their independence, all of which is likely to be more expensive for the welfare services in the long run. Yet there is also no doubt that – if people are able to stay put at home – they will need some support to do so, and this isn't straightforward.

All my older relations – aunts, cousins, and my mother – balked at the thought of having work done at home. My mother lived without central heating in her flat because she couldn't bear the thought of the men coming to put it in. She even had a danger notice put on her gas fire – her only source of warmth in the room in which she sat almost all day, every day – because she refused to have it replaced, or even serviced, for twenty years or so.

That is very common. So what should we do about it when we become old ourselves? Assume that we will be different? But we will be exactly the same. I already blanch at the thought of major building works, and I can completely see why my frail mother refused to go through with repairs. You can see why it is sometimes difficult to keep older people functioning in their homes, but the real problem is that the services we need to stay living at home are often simply not there. Where are the repair people who specialize in doing repairs for vulnerable older people? Where is the 'man with a van' who does minor jobs? There are some, but not many, and they tend to be supported by scarce grants. Families can do some of it, but what about those who have no family – or, at least, have no family nearby?

My mother used to say it wasn't worth putting in a new gas heater. 'I'm not going to live that long,' she would say.

I used to reply: 'What are you going to do? Freeze to death?'

The point is that people need and want to stay at home – or in the same vicinity – as long as they possibly can, but they are so often denied it because the right services are non-existent or the right kind of homes have never been built nearby. Everything I have discovered about ageing in the UK now, set out in the chapters before this one, makes it clear that life in old age can be real fun and utterly fulfilling, despite the gloomy news coverage and the agonizing media campaigns about dignity in hospital and in care homes. But so much of that depends on how people manage their changing needs for accommodation, so they can stay somewhere familiar, near familiar people and the networks that sustain them.

I have quoted the conclusion of the Joseph Rowntree Foundation's excellent report *From Welfare to Well-being* before, because it offers a fundamental insight into what is going wrong in so many aspects of ageing in the UK. 'Britain is still locked into a traditional welfare rationing approach for people on low incomes,' they argue, 'rather than a broader approach that applies to older people across all economic groups as citizens and consumers, and which draws in the private sector as partners.'[1]

They are right that our society has still not come to terms with the fact that we are an ageing society. Public services still focus, by and large, on the most vulnerable older people at times of crisis – perhaps 15 per cent of the older population – rather than adopting an approach which would allow the other 85 per cent to stay independent for as long as possible, to live their lives to the full – and to do so, as far as possible, at home.

It is hardly surprising to discover that, except in Wales, there is no overall government vision and strategy to plan for an ageing society. When Rowntree call for 'a new vision and culture ... at national, regional and local government levels, which celebrate older age and recognize the value of older people in society both individually and as a whole', they are criticizing a system that is – except in a crisis – blind to the needs of older people.

This chapter looks at the implications of this for the business of staying put, why we are making it so difficult for older people to do so, and why they find themselves mouldering in care homes far earlier than they need to.

One of the key trends in ageing in the UK is that older people – like the rest of society – increasingly live by themselves. Three in five women aged 75 and over live alone, whereas less than a third of the men of that age do. Very few of them live with anyone else, except partners or children, of course: only around three per cent. It is impossible to tell from the census whether this three per cent are in some kind of 'communes' of shared interests, or live together just for convenience and support, which is rare, or in some kind of residential care.

By far the largest number of these are over 90, probably mainly in care homes or nursing homes, down by a fifth over the decade for men and more than a third for women. It also isn't clear whether they are living alone instead because they can get support to do so, or because they are healthier. But so much of that depends on how they, as individuals and groups, and we as a society, manage their changing needs.

Those who do carry on living at home are mainly owner-occupiers, but that proportion goes down with age – from 79 per cent in the 50–64 age group, to 29 per cent of those who are 85 and older. Oddly enough, people's marital status also affects their housing circumstances. Widowed, married and single older households are more likely to live in homes they own outright, whilst divorced or separated people are more likely to live in social rented property.

Much more worrying – and the heart of the problem – is that a third of older households live in 'non-decent housing' (2001 figures) and that proportion goes up with age, and the worst cases tend to be renting in the private sector.

There is also a wide variation in the way that older people plan ahead. Some people really do so, whilst others don't believe that older age, and less independent older age in particular, will ever come to them. Some anticipate changes and plan accordingly whilst others find that income and access to capital can limit their choices. Still others find the choices on offer unacceptable, and refuse to choose at all.

One truly startling aspect of all this is just how many older people are faced with this array of unacceptable choices. Do you want to stay in your home, which is inadequately heated, which you can't afford to heat, and where maintenance levels are very low and you can't afford to have the work done that you need? Or even if you can afford it, you can't find someone reliable to do the job, who will come when he says he will, and treat you fairly. Or would you rather go into a nursing home where you will not have the privacy you crave and you can't take your pet cat? Where the food may well be terrible but at least you will be warm. What kind of choice is that? And why do we let older people face such choices when a little imagination and better forward planning could make such a difference?

There is already a major shift away from residential and nursing home type care to care in people's own homes, though it is often with inadequate support for the older people concerned. Unless they are fully mentally competent, very energetic and driven, it can be difficult to make sure all these fragmented services that are supposed to support them are co-ordinated at all.

Even then, Rowntree says that much of this shift from residential and nursing home care to people's own homes is not really a shift from a 'dependency' model to a 'promoting independence' approach. It is driven by a narrow risk-assessment model, rather than finding a solution that suits people best. Rowntree want both providers and commissioners of services – presumably including older people themselves – to use a quality of life assessment system, to decide on housing solutions according to what will be most life-enhancing. At the moment, decisions are often taken according to whether they will protect people from accidents, or – to be more accurate – protect professionals from getting the blame for accidents.

On that miserably narrow basis, the future lives of older people are determined.

Heating and repairs

The reason so many of those homes are 'non-decent', to use the jargon, is that they have inadequate heating. This is, in itself, the cause of one of the major scandals about the way older people are treated in modern society: between 20,000 and 50,000 older people die every winter because of the cold.

Usually the reasons for this cold are a lack of central heating – as many as 22 per cent of the households of people over 75 have no central heating – or they have poor-quality, badly maintained or ancient central heating systems. The older a household is, the less likely it is to be adequately heated or insulated, so that more than a third of households with someone over 85 fail on this standard.

There is official action on this, but the ability to make a difference is hampered by conflicting government targets. The Department for Business, Enterprise and Regulatory Reform (DBERR) restated the government's aim to eradicate fuel poverty in December 2007, making it clear it still wanted to eradicate fuel poverty in vulnerable households by 2010, with the proviso 'as far as reasonably practicable'.[2] Meanwhile, the Department for Communities' Decent Home Standard was set for the social housing sector, and aims to get 95 per cent of all social housing to meet a decent standard by 2010. Yet despite the target being expanded back in 2002 to cover all vulnerable households in the private sector, this is extraordinarily hard to achieve. The Department for Communities set a target of 70 per cent in the private sector by 2010, yet older people overwhelmingly live in private homes. So the state of their accommodation is not being targeted by one government department at the same rate that their fuel poverty is being targeted by DBERR.

Other reasons housing is thought to be non-decent include lack of maintenance and repairs, and lack of general modernization. Nor is this necessarily class or wealth related. It is more to do with age and not wanting the 'bother' of maintenance works than anything else. As I said, all my older relatives refused to have work done. Getting that work done depends, so often, on there being supportive family to make sure it happens and to manage the work, and move relatives in and out while work is going on. But supportive relatives are a luxury not every older person has.

If you look more closely at minority communities, the picture is even worse. One study in Leeds in 2004 among Afro-Caribbean older people found they had very little knowledge about renovation or repair grants, or the local city council Care and Repair scheme.[3] Even more extraordinary was that absolutely none of the interviewees received domiciliary care, meals on wheels or home help from the local social services.

These are often people who arrived in the UK to poor accommodation in the 1950s and 1960s, often living in overcrowded lodging houses with shared facilities and experiencing discrimination as well, who now find themselves back in a similarly powerless position. This phenomenon is repeated time and again amongst minority groups of older people, who are so often excluded from whatever help is available to the wider community of older people in any given area.

Back in 1992, the sociologist Malcolm Harrison looked at housing for black and minority ethnic communities, also in Leeds, and found an astonishing insensitivity to the various needs of different groups, often dressed up as an over-emphasis on cultural sensitivities – as if people from minority groups might not need security and good design, or as if their families might be wholly reliable carers.[4]

Thirteen years later, he warned again that: 'It is important to avoid stereotypes about the needs of elders or disabled people ... policy-makers should be wary of over-estimating the preparedness of service users' relatives to provide informal care ... people may be "left out" of kinship arrangements ... lack of explicit demand for a service will not necessarily imply absence of need, since problems of communication or cultural insensitivity of provision may diminish take-up.'[5]

It became horribly clear to me, as I did the research for this book, just how little thought goes into planning housing for older people, not just for minority groups but for everyone. As the Rowntree report showed, there is some thought about what the minority of older people who need serious help might require, but almost nothing about the rest of them. It is hardly surprising then that – for the want of the equivalent of a horseshoe nail – many of them have to leave their own homes, often at great expense to social services and at great personal distress.

If we took Rowntree's advice, we would not look just at housing for that tiny of minority of older people who live in sheltered-type housing. We would look instead much more broadly at:

- managing housing design so that it supports independence, but has easy access to adaptations and assistive technology to support ageing in one's own home
- getting flexible support into the home
- joining up housing services with health and care in order to create integrated teams in every neighbourhood.

Nor is this pleading with the government for more public spending. This investment will almost certainly save public money – if the adaptations were available, if there were local handyperson schemes, and if there were flexible and humane support services you could call on locally. But, as Rowntree said in 2003, these exist, they just tend to be fragmented and occasional much-praised one-off examples. They are certainly not the norm. Our manifesto, and the grey power activists who could use it, will certainly need to campaign for these services for the whole older and otherwise disabled population.

Improvement services

It is hardly surprising these services are so fragmented, because the funding available is barely sane. John Belcher, chief executive of Anchor Housing, the largest not-for-profit provider of housing, care and support for older people in England, has made a special demand that this mess should be sorted out. Anchor is the largest sole provider of Home Improvement Agency services in England, which are absolutely vital for many older people. But its Staying Put division is funded by Supporting People grants for poor older people, a very complex, time-consuming and uncertain funding stream, and some private-sector grants from the local authority, as well as earned fee income.

Belcher argues that a typical Home Improvement Agency would have about 30–35 per cent Supporting People funding, 20–25 per cent local authority funding, and a mere 6–10 per cent social service or health funding, with the rest coming from charitable sources and earned fee income.

One solution would be for these Home Improvement Agencies to broaden their work to include private work for older clients, as some of them are beginning to do. In fact, there would be an enormous demand for this kind of service, because most older people want to know that the work is being done under supervision –

rather than relying on someone who has put a card through their door – so that they can trust those who are doing it, and they have some comeback if it is not satisfactory.

Anchor and its colleagues and competitors could really add to the security of older people by providing this service on an earned fee basis. That would, in itself, begin to move provision away from the seat-of-the-pants welfare model to a more general provision, with additional funding for the poorest.

Adaptations at home

Whether they plan ahead or not, relatively few people have adaptations done to their homes once physical frailty sets in, and, when they do, it is often when a crisis occurs. The oldest age groups are obviously the most likely to need those adaptations, especially those in the poorest health, yet when the crisis happens it often takes ages to get the adaptations made, whether the individuals are able to pay for them or not.

This is truly ridiculous. It would save local authorities money if they had a team of people who could just get the adaptations done quickly. Even the assessment process would save money, if they could speed it up – just by getting those who fit the adaptations to do the assessments – because delays often mean that these older people will end up in a care home, costing the council far more. Even if people can afford to pay for the adaptations, they often need information, advice and support before getting the work done, and it would be sensible for local authorities – who carry out the adaptations for those unable to pay – and for those in social and council housing to offer that support to those who can pay as well. But that will only help if the local authorities can themselves speed up the process of doing the assessments and helping people find the right workmen to carry out the work, supervise it – if necessary, taking a handling fee – and check that the adaptation serves its purpose for the older person concerned.

Some wealthier older people might also plan to move into retirement housing either for rent or for sale in the future. They also need information, support and help in making choices. Some of them are in groups who are loosely described as being at the greatest risk, especially women over 80, whose social networks tend to be shrinking, living alone and without children.

As far as rental is concerned, some of the key people who might think about moving to sheltered accommodation are those living in run-down neighbourhoods like Chapeltown in Leeds, who have limited or no alternatives – just the people who need the information provided for them.

When the International Longevity Centre carried out research into this problem, asking people what kind of changes they might need to their own homes as they got older, they found that people consistently underestimated what they would need.[6] They need advice, yet what local advice there is tends to be achingly slow and restricted to the poorest.

Moving house

There is no doubt that older people tend to avoid moving house if they possibly can. Owner-occupiers over the age of 70 are the least likely to move voluntarily, closely followed by older people in social class E, who are the least likely to want to move, even though they often complain most about their neighbourhood. If older people do plan to move, it is often to be nearer family and friends.

But there is a contradiction about where they move to that underlines how frustrating it can be. Sheltered housing is more acceptable to social classes ABC1, but they tend not to live in sheltered housing anyway. Those who actually use it are drawn proportionately more from groups D and E, who are not nearly so keen on the idea. Data on the people who live in sheltered housing now suggest that, if we want more older people living there – possibly with extra care – then the standards need to be very high. A great deal of practical information also needs to be made available to potential residents to get them to show an interest at all, let alone make the decision to take up the offer of a place in sheltered housing when it becomes available.

What planners and policy-makers don't seem to understand is that, as people get older, their homes become more and more important to them. This ought to be fairly obvious: as you get older and frailer, you tend to be in your own home more of the time, so of course it becomes even more important to you than before. Also, if your memory is frail, even before full-blown dementia, then the familiar is easier than the new. Home surroundings where you have lived for many years are easier to negotiate. Even when the dementia has developed, people can often still find their way around surroundings they have known all their lives.

It is hardly surprising, therefore, that 82 per cent of older people want to stay in their own homes. If that is impossible, they have a variety of different preferences. A small proportion, those who are better off, might move to purpose-built or supported housing where higher levels of need can be met. There are now several companies providing schemes like that, which are relatively expensive but quite popular with those who can afford them.

This isn't an option for most people, especially because as they get older they regard their home less and less as a financial resource, available to release equity when they need it. Most people realize that they may need to sell their homes, if they own them, to pay for care at the end of life, but that is considerably resented, both by the older people themselves and by their children, particularly where it affects one partner in a relationship. It isn't usually regarded as a good option when it comes to paying for more suitable accommodation.

But all this assumes that older people will have thought ahead about what to do when the time comes. Help the Aged published a report in 2006 which showed that two thirds of baby boomers had made no plans for their future care needs.[7] In fact, the survey found widespread confusion among those approaching retirement age about what would happen to them. Almost half believed that the government would contribute in some way towards their care needs, with one in ten 61–65 year olds optimistically believing the state would pick up the bill for all their future care.

Well over half (55 per cent) believed that, if they needed a place in a care home one day, their basic state pension (£84) would be one way to cover the £400 a week average cost. A similar proportion thought their personal savings would be enough, despite two in three not having made any plans for anticipated care costs. One in five people said they expected to rely on help from their relatives to pay their care bills, presumably their children. You have to wonder how they manage to budget for the rest of their lives.

Help the Aged has been warning consistently that the public's care-free attitudes towards their future needs, combined with the government's unfair and complex care system, have resulted in thousands of pensioners not getting the care they desperately need. Help the Aged's senior policy manager, Jonathan Ellis, warned that:

> *Views held by society that ageing is something that should be feared are perpetuated even further by a care funding system that no one can understand. It is apparent that the*

public have been led into a false sense of security about
what is, and what is not, available to help them if they
have care needs. Many people feel let down by the very
system meant to help them. It is understandable that they
should question why they worked hard to save, only to
have those savings taken from them if they are
unfortunate enough to develop care needs. If the
government is serious about tackling the care funding
crisis, it needs to invest more in care services, and help
people to plan ahead for future care needs.

Help the Aged has clearly got an agenda here. It wants the government to end the complex and undignified means-testing system, which forces many older people to sell their homes to meet care costs. It also wants an increase in the upper savings limits. Currently, if you have savings of £21,000 or more (England and NI, not Scotland and Wales), including the value of your home, you are expected to meet the full cost of your care home fees without any state funding.

It also wants a doubling of the level of personal expense allowance, from £19.60 per week, to £40. This is the money that a local council will leave you with when deciding how much it will take from you to fund care provided in a care home. As well as this, and applying much more generally to all this debate, it is calling for the NHS to introduce a single, national assessment process to decide who should receive fully funded NHS care.

That is still a long way away, presumably because clarity would mean more calls on the public purse, which funders want to choke off where possible, though it is specifically very frail older people who are suffering. The Department of Health launched a consultation in summer 2006 on a new framework for continuing care (also known as fully funded NHS care). Its key aim was to propose clear national policies for eligibility and assessment processes, which would get rid of the 'postcode lottery', but there is no change as yet.

Help the Aged also wants to see a change in the boundary between what is defined as 'health' and what is 'social care', such as help with washing, dressing or taking daily medication, which has caused a great deal of confusion for years. Decisions about who is eligible for social care services are taken by local councils, who also decide how much people should pay towards those services. This has led to major differences from one area to the next as to what will and what will not be provided by the state. Unfortunately, the NHS funding system is no clearer. The NHS is legally required to pay for care where a person's primary need is for health care, but every health authority has different criteria for what constitutes a 'health need'.

It is hardly surprising it is so confusing, and – because it is confusing – there is very little encouragement to plan ahead, or even think much about the effect that housing can have on our health and well-being when we are older. Then, when the crisis happens – a fall or accident at home – it is too late to think carefully. Younger people certainly need to put some thought into how they want to live, how they can plan ahead to stay put at home. But care providers are going to have to think much more carefully about what older people actually want and how to provide it, or at least how to make what is available more attractive – and what services people will need to help them stay independent. In the meantime, older people themselves will have to campaign for the kinds of accommodation they want to see, if they can't stay at home.

Housing choice

The truth about what is available now is that there is very little choice, particularly in public housing services, which include local authorities and housing associations. People certainly don't feel they have choices, even when they do, and those who can afford to buy or rent in the private sector may well not do so because they have little information and even less sense of what choices are before them.

So the builders, housing providers and public and voluntary sectors all have a huge task ahead of them in finding out what people really want as they get older, trying to match their offering to that, and then learning how to provide the support people need at home in order to stay there.

Satellite schemes from sheltered housing have been in operation for years with mixed success. A few older people have tried setting up a 'commune style' environment, buying a big house, converting it and sharing staff, something which is pretty widespread in Europe and the USA. Some extra care provision in sheltered housing has allowed people to stay in the same place and die there, but that is fairly rare: usually when people get sick they get sent to hospital, even if they don't want to be. There are a few retirement villages – there are far more in the USA – but they do not seem to have caught the imagination of older people over here.

So something is seriously wrong here. It isn't that somehow the providers have made a mistake about what older people want, it's that they haven't even thought it was important to find out. So the combination of independence and choice that so many older people actually want is ever more elusive. Once again, it is going to have to be older people who launch a vigorous and aggressive campaign for the right to real choice of home and care for themselves. Until they do so, it will probably remain just as elusive.

Lifetime homes

When the Joseph Rowntree Foundation carried out a literature review on housing with care in later life in 2006, they confirmed that independence and security were what most older people wanted, but found that residents and housing providers interpreted 'independence' rather differently.[8] Nor is it clear whether housing with care actually keeps people embedded in social networks. Many people do find greater opportunities for social interaction, but people with physical, cognitive and sensory impairments are consistently identified in all the studies as 'being on the margins of social groups and networks, and in some cases the focus of hostility'.

Nor does housing with care always seem to work as an alternative to residential or nursing home care, because people often still move on to that – for a variety of reasons, including increasing care needs and their own or their relatives' preference for something different, or something that provided more care generally. There is also worrying evidence about whether housing with care provides enough support for people with severe dementia, most of whom will end up in residential or nursing homes. Despite the publicity and promotional material for such schemes, which tend to suggest that they offer 'a home for life', the term is open to wide interpretation.

Only one scheme in the Rowntree survey, which has its own onsite care home, came anywhere near offering a 'home for life', albeit within the boundaries of the scheme rather than in the residents' own homes. Nor did any of the studies they reviewed look at the issue of the end of life, nor how palliative care services have been, or might be, integrated into care provision.

The idea of 'lifetime homes', which can really be adapted as their residents get older, has not yet taken root in the UK, despite being popular in other countries. Conservative leader David Cameron argued in 2006 that the UK should invest in such housing, which is a good sign.[9] Rowntree estimated that lifetime homes would save taxpayers some £5.5 billion over 60 years by reducing the need for adaptations to existing houses, and by allowing people to stay in their own homes rather than move to care homes. But the Home Builders Federation has argued that 'the whole concept of lifetime houses is a waste of resources' because too few older people stayed in their own homes.

We are caught in a Catch-22 here, because older people don't stay simply because their homes are unsuitable. We need builders with vision to take on the challenge. The additions would not cost much, according to Gary Day of McCarthy & Stone, one of the largest builders of private retirement homes, 'the little simple touches to a new-build, such as easy-turn taps, light sockets at a convenient height, or eye level ovens. It's the infrastructure that is expensive.'[10] The government has listened closely to this concern and recently published its paper 'Lifetime Homes, Lifetime Neighbourhoods: A National Strategy for Housing in an Ageing Society',[11] which attempts to ensure that all new-built housing will cope with disabilities and be wheelchair-friendly.

The remarkable Jewish Community Housing for the Elderly project in the USA, which is actually a mixture of Jewish, Russian and Chinese, has been trying to make a difference to the end of life of their residents. They have a nurse available and a sick bay, and have tried, as far as it was possible, to keep dying residents at home, even though the place was not truly geared up for it. But in the UK, housing with care schemes have barely begun to think about what it means genuinely to provide 'homes for life'.

Anything worthy of the name of a 'home for life' should be exactly that. It should include the possibility of palliative care being provided right there on site. Everyone accepts there will be accidents and illnesses which will require a trip to hospital, but if people move into an extra care provider's flat, they ought to be allowed to die there.

Ghettoization

Then we have to settle the perennial question of whether schemes work best when they are mixed, with the fitter and the frailer, physically and mentally, living together, or whether it is better to provide services just for the very frail. This is another area where older people are going to have to confront the providers, because many providers – particularly those in the voluntary sector – provide only for one section of the community, for Asian elders for instance, or for African-Caribbeans.

The housing provided tends to be for the less well-off, the majority of those in sheltered housing often having got there because they used to live in a registered social landlord's property. There is Jewish Sheltered Housing, or Methodist Homes for the Aged, or the Paddington Churches Housing Association, all originally designed for one section of the community, and all to some extent opening out beyond it.

But it is peculiarly narrow to imagine that this is really acceptable. Although most of us might choose to live where there are lots of people of similar backgrounds, there is no virtue in deliberate ghettoization. It is bad enough to be ghettoized by age, with retirement villages for the old, or sheltered housing or residential care.

To add to that a further narrowing of entry seems to distance such places and institutions even further from the real world without actually becoming closed communities.

Is that what people really want? Or has it grown up, just as the same 'welfare-style' thinking has brought us hostels for people who have a history of mental illness, or special housing for ex-offenders? Isn't it far more likely that this is design by social 'problem' group rather than by residents' preferences, perhaps because that is how the funding is organized? Isn't it actually planned just to make it easier for the staff?

American experience suggests that we can have supported housing, as they do there, for people with mental health problems, older people, people with full-blown AIDS and ex-offenders all living close to each other. Jewish Community Housing in Boston is open to all sorts of groups, Jewish and non-Jewish alike, but with a Jewish flavour. Why not a Chinese or Asian flavour? There is no reason why we have to perpetuate the UK model – so divorced from real life that the phrase 'care in the community' is a joke – of older people's ghettos or, as you find so often, exclusively Jewish residents cared for by entirely non-Jewish staff, usually black.

New models

When senior nurse Nikki Lewis got fed up with finding somewhere decent for her father to retire to, she decided to build somewhere herself, and turned a former Dorset prep school into two- and three-bedroom apartments. There is another retirement village taking shape in Ditchling in Sussex, to be operated by a religious order, with 232 independent living units and 180 long-term care beds, and the core of the village will include a café, restaurants, a swimming pool and various meeting places as well as a shop. Both are following in the footsteps of Hartrigg Oaks, just outside York, developed by the Joseph Rowntree Housing Trust, with independent living in bungalows, where support can be provided, with extra care sheltered housing around a central site, with a 42 bed care home for short-term respite or where residents can live out the ends of their lives.

All these raise questions about how much people will want to live exclusively with other older people. There was also a problem at Hartrigg Oaks about people who needed better facilities for dementia.[12] But these new communities are the result of thinking about helping people stay in their own homes even when they are seriously ill. Even so, I have wondered about whether people can really stay there until they actually die. The American models have avoided ghettoization, at least as far as providing two- or three-bedroomed flats, so that grandchildren and others can visit. But can people actually die there?

Care villages may not quite be a 'home for life', and other models around the world suggest that they may not have facilities for palliative care at the end. But they are a possible model and, although the service charges are high, they don't cost as much as residential care.

There is another model beginning to emerge which I believe will turn out to be even more important: a commune-style housing solution, which encourages residents to provide mutual support for each other when social services are in short supply. One key example of this is the Vivarium project in Scotland, supported by two universities, and described in the *Glasgow Herald* as a 'futuristic commune for older people, the first project of its kind in the country'.[13]

Vivarium includes plans for 20 to 30 homes, a shared kitchen and lounge for socializing, bulk-buying of food to cut costs, co-owned cars, and even a hot tub. The baby boom generation behind the scheme were young when hippie communes became fashionable in the 1960s. The name itself is tongue in cheek: it means a glass tank for reptiles.

This kind of project is now known as 'co-housing', resident-managed communities with a mix of independent and shared living space, and they are becoming more common in Denmark, New Zealand and the Netherlands. Most are quite 'green', though by no means all, but it is this model of shared space plus privacy that seems to hold considerable attractions for a great many older people, particularly if it can be managed so that care can be provided if needed, formally or informally.

'It really started with a couple of us sitting thinking old age is not an attractive proposition and we realized we did not like the options available at present and thought, "We will have to change them",' said Vivarium founder Anne Pattullo. She persuaded the Royal Bank of Scotland Centre for the Older Person's Agenda at Queen Margaret University College in Edinburgh to conduct a feasibility study, to look at the capital required, how homes could be owned or leased and what could happen when residents die or leave. The Sustainability Centre at Glasgow Caledonian University wants to be involved too, and Age Concern Scotland has given £500 towards administration costs. Fife Council and NHS Fife are also taking an interest.

'This group is not accepting the status quo of housing we provide for them, of always being passive and saying "it is sheltered housing or care",' said QMUC research manager Belinda Dewar. 'They are about being proactive and thinking now about what they would like for the future. I think other older people can listen to that story and think it is possible for them as well.'

Co-housing has particularly taken off in the Netherlands, where there are at least 200 projects and the government is prepared to invest. They expect older people in co-housing to make reduced use of health and social services because they will be happier and healthier. It is also emerging in the USA, where older people can stay in one home for the remainder of their lives, relying on the support of good friends who are neighbours, on-site co-operative healthcare and a hospice for the very end. Like Glacier Circle in Davis, California, where twelve old friends (average age: 80) found and bought land together, hired an architect, ironed out insurance together and now have exactly what they wanted – individual town houses grouped round a courtyard, with a 'common house' with large kitchen and dining room for communal dinner, and living room. Upstairs are studio apartments they will rent at below market value to skilled nurses who will provide extra care.

But in the UK co-housing is still the preserve of determined groups of older people with visions of a different choice of living, like the Older Women's CoHousing Project (Owch), a group of two dozen Londoners aged between 51 and 81 which is looking for a property that would provide them each with a separate flat as well as a shared laundry, community space and other communal quarters.[14] Although the group has been in existence for some eight years, and it meets monthly to discuss progress, it still hasn't (at least when we went to press) found a suitable property. The Housing Corporation has begun to show some interest, but the UK is still decades behind other countries.

Call to arms

Policy-makers explain that older people are choosing new solutions for their housing, but the truth is that actually they have no idea, because there is hardly any choice at all at the moment. While in other countries, like the Netherlands and the USA, entrepreneurs and social innovators have pressed ahead with a range of new kinds of housing, very few have come forward in the UK.

Consequently older people have to make do with what there is: their own homes, without adaptation or modernization or access to reliable builders, let alone proper day-to-day home care. Alternatively, they can move away to a 'retirement village', cut off from the real world, or sheltered accommodation with the prospect of another move all too soon. Or they face the dependence of a residential or care home.

A very small number of people have developed something different for themselves, borrowing from some of the techniques of mutual support from the USA and of mutual housing – to carry on being with their friends all the way through. This co-housing idea has enormous potential for older people, and the fact that it remains so difficult in this country is part of the tragedy for older people in our society, whether because mutualism makes officials nervous or because they simply never consider the aspirations of older people anyway.

So a key part of our manifesto should demand this. **Entrepreneurs, policy-makers, charitable foundations and planners, along with those who are campaigning for this, must develop a usable co-housing package that can be adapted by groups of friends and other organizations to house themselves affordably, provide each other with mutual support, with the people they choose and for as long as they want.**

It really is extraordinary that co-housing should be so difficult here, especially as people are agitating for it. Part of the problem is that housing associations have become sclerotic adjuncts to the Housing Corporation, rather than the brave, experimental and responsive organizations – part of the voluntary sector – that we need. We need to re-invent them, set them free from the straitjacket that forces them to hand over nomination rights to new homes to the local authority, and let them spin off experimental organizations that imaginative people can invest in, and allow them to find new solutions for staying put when they are older.

The manifesto also needs to include demands to:

- **Insist that a 'home for life' is just that.** That means that sheltered housing has to extend to palliative care and proper care for people with dementia. It is time that older people were given a real choice about where they are to live.

- **Build houses and ground-floor flats so that they can be adapted easily for older people to provide them with genuinely lifetime homes, which can accommodate them until they die.** My mother lived in an older block of flats, and it really isn't beyond the wit of freeholders and local authorities to make sure that six or eight of them should eventually become the equivalent of sheltered housing, with a wheelchair ramp at the back.

- **Provide sheltered housing, with nursing care, and co-housing options in every neighbourhood.** Why should we expect older people to move away from everything and everyone familiar when they get older, when moving is most traumatic – and then expect them to move again because there are no facilities for nursing them at home either.

- **Provide a nationwide local network of handyperson services which specialize in repair work for older people.** This is an obvious job for the big older people's charities, working with local authorities. But local authorities have to respond as well, creating local teams that bring together housing, health and social care. Another solution would be for these Home Improvement Agencies to broaden their work to include private work for older clients, as some of them are beginning to do so.

- **Insist that local authorities provide proper advice about housing options for older people.** There is almost no comprehensive information available at the moment, either about what is available or about the costs involved. And if this is beyond local authorities, it surely isn't beyond the wit of the world of the internet to provide some kind of national housing and care service for older people online.

Chapter 7

Don't treat those who look after me like rubbish

Train and reward care assistants properly

My family has been to hell and back. The care my mother received in a home has disgusted us. She was dirty, neglected and ill-treated by staff who deprived her of water and served her packet soup without noticing that she had the wrong cutlery to eat it with.

Mrs M, *What Price Care in Old Age?* Spain coalition, 2005

You could say that putting someone in a bed with cot sides so they can't get out is assault, it's imprisoning them, it would be considered assault if it was done to you or me, but if it's done to an 80-year-old with dementia, it's considered ordinary.

Alison Clarke, *Showing Restraint*, Counsel and Care, 2002

I had a letter while I was researching this book from Dee Sedgwick, whose mother had been a resident at a care home in the south of England run by a well-known insurance company.[1] For the first two years, the care she received was not too bad, but when her dementia became serious, the problems began.

'The level of care diminished on a sliding scale to the increasing severity of Mum's mental frailty,' Dee wrote. 'My husband and I ... visited Mum on a daily basis, at different times of the day. On almost every occasion (we tried to go along at meal times) her food and drink were out of reach with no "care" worker assisting Mum with her meal. However, during the last few months, Mum actually needed to be fed, like a baby, and that wasn't happening.'

They tried to complain and received various reassurances. Then her mother was rushed to hospital with severe dehydration, malnutrition and rotting, necrotizing bedsores. The managers denied the presence of these bedsores until Dee finally got evidence from the local district nurses, who knew also that they could be aggravated by malnutrition. Her mother was put on a drip to rehydrate her, but the damage had been done and her internal organs had been ruined from 'the deprivation of fluid and food in an 82-year-old lady'.

This is just one of a whole catalogue of shocking stories about care homes for older people which emerge every year. The treatment wasn't deliberate cruelty – though there are examples of Dickensian conditions and continuing abuse which might as well be deliberate, as we shall see – but it was an example of something else which is almost as shocking: a thoughtless, unimaginative and inhuman approach to caring for older people, simply because they are old.

Cruelty is nothing new, but there are underlying reasons – not the least of which is plummeting financial support for care – why this is turning into such a crisis now, and why the word 'care' has become so perverted.

There is a yawning gap between official policy and what actually happens in reality to older individuals, who – simply because they are old – are less interesting to the media, and less of a concern to politicians. We congratulate ourselves on our enlightened policies to provide people with the care they need so that they can stay in their own homes as they get older, but blind ourselves to the meagre and fast-disappearing care that is available. We congratulate ourselves on our policies to pay for personal care, even if it is just for the poorest, but blind ourselves to the fact that it is delivered by untrained people, who are paid abominably, and are themselves bullied by penny-pinching, technocratic management regimes.

Care is an absolutely vital part of any manifesto. It enables older people to live independently for longer. It potentially saves the welfare services a great deal of money. If it is poor, inhuman or absent, then none of those things are possible.

Care provision

The debate at the heart of care is about what kind of care we will need in the future. The number of people in traditional care homes has been falling for a decade, and is now below half a million people. This may be because older people shun the very idea, but it is also partly because of government cuts in payment for care homes. Anything up to 600 care homes are now closing every year, with devastating consequences for those who live in them. This may not be a sign of reducing demand at all. In fact, the Government Actuary is predicting a tripling in the volume of demand to 1.2 million residents by 2051.

Recent reports have warned that, though some of that demand can be met with home care and extra care services, we need to rebuild the traditional care home sector as well. But the Department of Health disagrees, arguing that older people now want something different. Both sides are right about some aspects of the argument, but – behind the polite policy debate – older people are getting seriously angry. And if you read the 2005 King's Fund report on *The Business of Caring*, you can see why.[2]

They found good services everywhere, but also inflexible services which never listen, and 'situations where, frankly, the promise of choice or control seems very hollow'. Their conclusions were that people actually have limited choice and control over what they get, and are being put at risk from untrained and unqualified staff.

The King's Fund was looking at the situation in London, where property prices are high, so operators often close their care homes at short notice, and where funding is in short supply. They often have rigid 15 or 30 minute visiting rules and high staff turnover, so that vulnerable older people don't get to know their carers, many of whom speak poor English, and get inadequate services. It is not a pretty picture, and when it comes to care homes the majority of London authorities 'export' their older people to become residents in outer London boroughs or beyond, which means that, if they have friends or family, it becomes even harder for them to stay in touch. But then this is, of course, cheaper.

The funding of care home places is also increasingly obscure, with Scotland running an entirely different system, and evidence that the NHS has virtually stopped paying care home bills in large areas of Britain. There are 40 primary care trusts (PCTs) where the NHS meets bills for those who need intensive nursing in care home places for only one in every 10,000 residents. There are five that fund care home bills for just one in 20,000 of their local populations. The Department of Health acknowledged in 2004 that 'the system has been difficult for older people and their families, which is why we are consulting on this issue to simplify it'. But a generous, nationally consistent system still seems a long way away.

Technically, the NHS has a duty to pay for those who meet stringent tests of their level of medical need. But people in care homes who don't qualify must pay their own bills, unless they have very little in the way of savings or assets and can pass a tough means test applied by social workers – who are often under instruction to be as tough as possible. There has been a series of test cases, as well as a highly critical report from the Health Service Ombudsman, highlighting unfairness in decision making and obscure guidance from the Department of Health, as well as a sense that there was something arbitrary and inconsistent about the way the system was working.[3] But none of this seems to have made NHS trusts more generous with their funding, and that is why the Department of Health has been trying to set new national standards about who qualifies for NHS aid, in order to replace local assessments, which are constantly challenged. But unless there is a great deal more money available, the chances are that national criteria will mean that the rules will be drawn even tighter, and even more older people will be denied help.

This is a storm which has been gathering for some time. A coalition of older people's charities, including Age Concern and Help the Aged, formed an alliance called Spain (Social Policy on Ageing Information Network). Spain's investigation found that local authorities are still paying lower rates for older people's residential care than for other groups – in 2004, local authorities were only prepared to pay an average of £377 for older people, while younger adults were offered £447 to £734.[4]

They heard from many older people distressed about living in dirty housing, waiting months for a bath or being trapped at home because they have no access to a basic wheelchair ramp or grab rail. Many 24-hour carers are forced to go without a break for months because there is not enough funding for respite. Older people also say the help they receive at home is rushed and they are not told when the visits will be. And carers reach the end of their tether, which is what leads them to collapse, or to abuse the people they care for – often someone they love dearly – and to reach desperation point. Then the person they are caring for goes into care, costing far more money than before.

'Social services don't seem to listen,' said Margaret Cracknell, whose husband has cerebral palsy and needs 24-hour care from her. 'No one helped us to get the help we needed. All they said was that my husband didn't want to spend any time in a home so he shouldn't have to go in. But no one took my feelings into account. I'm his carer – if I can't cope, he can't cope. Health professionals have told me that it's down to the money. There's not enough to go round so they keep you waiting in the system, hoping you'll go away. And that has happened to me.'[5]

Once again, the question is the extent to which this is a service model or really a welfare model, with others deciding – and assessing – what is suitable for an individual or a couple. Tony Robinson, the actor best known for his appearances in the Blackadder TV series, claims old people are in any case being treated as second-class citizens and that the allowances are just insufficient: 'It strikes me as quite extraordinary that if you foster a child you get up to £300 a week,' he said. 'If you are a carer, looking after someone who is elderly and infirm – sacrificing your life and your career for them – you get £45 a week.'[6]

The emerging crisis is below the media radar – old people are not news – and therefore largely below the government's antennae as well. But the effects are all too real. Take Miss Tugwell, for example: doubly incontinent, she has had the number of baths her carers can give her reduced from two a week to one, and they now say she may have to make do with being sponged down:

> *I feel unclean half the time. I felt deprived when social*
> *services cut me down from two to one bath a week in*
> *2004 – deprived of feeling like a normal adult. Then they*
> *told me I had to stop having the one bath a week I have*
> *now because my care was taking longer than the one*
> *hour I was allocated. I told them I was doubly incontinent*
> *and why on earth couldn't I have a bath? Wasn't I*
> *entitled to be properly clean? They told me that time and*
> *money wouldn't allow it. But we're talking about fifteen*
> *minutes.*[7]

After her protests, the council agreed to let her keep having one weekly bath. This was at the beginning of the *Observer*'s Dignity at Home campaign, and they are not the only ones campaigning against this quiet, insidious discrimination that affects the most powerless people of all. Yet the Local Government Association is forecasting that, by 2009, only people assessed as having 'critical' or 'substantial' needs will be eligible for support of any kind. The recent Commission for Social Care Inspection's scathing report found that seven out of ten local authorities now restrict help with basic care – dressing, washing and toileting – to very serious cases.[8]

There is talk in response of a hypothecated tax on inheritances below the tax threshold, which would fund care for older people and still only tax the average estate of £80,000 at £2,000. The author of that original proposal, Philip Spiers, managing director of the advisory Nursing Home Fees Agency, says that 'the yield would be instant, simple, and would keep track of demographic changes and inflation'. At the time of the Royal Commission, he thought it was difficult. He now thinks the time is right.

Meanwhile, Scotland has a different system of free personal care, put in place after the recommendations of the Royal Commission on Long Term Care 1997–9, chaired by a well-known Scot, Sir Stewart (now Lord) Sutherland, although government in England refused to back it and two commissioners dissented. Some people were afraid it would discourage informal care, but that hasn't happened. The problem in Scotland is that it cost much more than expected: £127 million in 2002/3 compared with the expected £17 million.

That has put increasing pressure on the system. The cuts are becoming more obvious, and people are kept waiting for assessments for longer. Three quarters of Scottish councils are struggling to cover the costs. One council, Renfrewshire, even used a debt collection agency to pursue the family of an 87-year-old dementia sufferer over a £500 bill for food preparation, which they said wasn't covered. By June 2006, almost 5,000 pensioners were on waiting lists for personal care across Scotland.

There is also a crisis in the private care home sector in Scotland over whether local authority payments per patient are enough. 'We just can't compete at the moment,' said Robert Kilgour, owner of Forth Care, which operates three homes in Edinburgh and two in Musselburgh. 'The council is looking to introduce more red tape. The money we get at the moment makes it really tight. And all the time property prices are continuing to rise, making it less and less profitable to stay open. I'm seriously considering closing all the homes I have in Edinburgh and redeveloping them for residential [use]. I know of several other nursing-home providers who are just as frustrated as me.'[9]

Care funding solutions

Both the funding for care and nursing homes and the funding for social care at home have taken a serious hit over recent years. The system is in chaos. The minister concerned, Ivan Lewis, described the state of adult social care as 'neither sustainable nor desirable'. It is so confusing and unfair that the King's Fund commissioned Sir Derek Wanless to produce a review of it all, called *Securing Good Care for Older People,* which was published in 2006.[10]

Wanless's proposals were a free package of the most basic care for everyone, but with extra services, defined and up to a maximum optimal package, which are co-funded by the state and the individual, with the state matching the individual's optional contributions pound for pound. The idea was that those on low incomes would make their optional co-payments though new means-tested benefits provided precisely for that purpose. The advantage of getting people to pay for an element themselves is that it acts as a kind of brake on people claiming more services than they need.

The Wanless solution is a kind of 'partnership model', which leads to the service becoming more universal because means testing, as such, would disappear from it, and it would also make the point that most people would have to pay for a part of their costs, which seems fair enough. The Wanless scheme would lead to additional public spending of about £4.2 billion, but some of that could be offset by a saving on non-means-tested benefits, reducing the public funding required by £2.5 billion.

All this needs to be set against evidence from the public about how they deal with the costs now. The Joseph Rowntree Foundation found that, for many people, the best strategy for funding their own long-term care appeared to be disposing of their assets in advance to make sure they qualified for state support.[11] The current means testing seems to encourage people to pass their money on to their children, or worse, a general fecklessness that sits poorly with any system that tries to be fair.

Rowntree's solution was, among other reforms, a voluntary equity release scheme for home-based care, so that home owners could access the capital tied up in their homes. It would cost some £100 million a year, but it would actually cost a fraction of that in the long run as the loans got repaid.

They also wanted to double the capital threshold for care home support, so that home owners did not feel they had to drain so much of the proceeds from their properties before accessing state support (cost: £250–300 million a year) and to double the personal expenses allowances for people supported by local authorities in care homes (cost: £250 million a year). This would make a huge difference to people who find it very hard to get all the services they want, such as podiatry, on the money they are left with.

Because they have to contribute to the costs of their care, people have to give up most of their pension payments to pay towards the fees. They are only entitled to retain a Personal Expenses Allowance of £19.60 per week, designed to cover the cost of all the personal items not covered by their care home fees 'on stationery, personal toiletries, treats and small presents', according to the NHS guidance. In practice, they often have to use this on other services like physiotherapy and chiropody which otherwise have long NHS waiting lists.

At one stage, the Rowntree Foundation was thinking of paying for some of this by charging all care home residents for the non-care costs and redistributing them, which would be very hard to justify. But their final proposal is absolutely critical: to review the basis of the present Attendance Allowance. Plenty of people who do not need it are getting it, whilst others truly struggle on. If nothing else happens, that certainly should: the present system is unfair, idio-syncratic, and doesn't always reach the people who need it most. The equity release option is already available to people with very valuable homes, but the idea of extending it to people with less valu-able properties is a good one.

In a previous book, *The Moral State We're In*, I suggested a dif-ferent model. Approximately one in four older people will need long-term care of some kind – which is so high that it might seem like the kind of risk we should expect people to take on for themselves, up to a point. Supposing the system asked older people to pay for some of the risk – perhaps the average long-term care period of two years – and then, if they needed longer, the state would pay. That kind of solution would have several virtues. First, it would deal with the unfairness issue: it is reasonable to ask people to save for the possibility of two years of long-term care, and the costs would not be limitless – people would not normally have to sell their home or give everything away. The difficulty would be calculating the start point, but that is not an impossible task.

Ministers have now promised an inquiry into the postcode lot-tery of care for older people. Ivan Lewis said that 'the rationing of services for frail and infirm people in England had become incon-sistent and unfair'.[12] He said increasing numbers of local authori-ties were imposing a vulnerability test to stop people getting help when their condition was not yet life threatening.

Without some kind of reform, services will continue to evapo-rate, though there is an increasing number of charities and coali-tions of organizations running campaigns to press for change, such as Counsel and Care, Carers UK and Help the Aged combining for their Right Care Right Deal campaign. Think-tanks like Demos say that the baby-boomer generation has been brought up to expect far more from services than their parents did, and will not put up with the current situation. In fact, they *are* doing so: neither they, nor their parents, who are experiencing these savage cuts and lack of availability, are actually making a fuss. In practice, instead of fighting it, they may just accept they are going to have to sell their homes to pay, unless some other arrangements are made.

Care homes

Without adequate care at home, most people will find that the only likely alternative is still a care home or nursing home, although the number of places is still falling. The Scottish crisis has its parallel around the rest of the UK, as families are often asked to pay top-up fees, even when the local authority is supposed to pay.

Part of the problem is that there is very little information available about local care homes, what they should reasonably cost and what the choices are. The Office of Fair Trading (OFT) has recommended that care homes should provide the price in writing of accommodation and residential or nursing fees before anyone enters the home. They should all have proper written contracts or statements of terms. Of course they should. The OFT was critical of the care home sector for its practice of charging 'top-up' fees, but it was also very critical of local authorities for failing to give families help and information, whether they were self-payers, funded by the local authority, or in the unenviable position of being funded by the local authority and being asked for a top-up by the care home operators of anything up to an extra £200 a week.

The OFT said that those at greatest risk of being 'cheated' were those who paid at least part of their own bills. They become vulnerable: they don't want to move when they are asked for a huge increase, and their family doesn't want to move them either. It often leaves them with little choice, and without a proper agreement and contract it amounts to a form of blackmail of vulnerable people.

But the practice is still going on. One local authority wrote regularly to people who were only vaguely associated with the person in care, like a neighbour who once collected their pension for them, demanding that they pay top-ups. Esme Collins, 103, was threatened with eviction from her privately run Abbeymoor nursing home in Worksop, Nottinghamshire, in 2007, unless she paid another £125 a week.[13] In her case, the minister intervened and the threat was lifted.

But the real problem is that block-buying of bed spaces in care homes by local authorities means that fees for individual places are distorted, and so the market does not operate freely. Often it means that the self-payers are, in effect, subsidizing the costs of those who are paid for by local authorities, which is hardly fair, let alone ethical. It also means that some care homes find themselves receiving large numbers of local-authority-funded older people, which means that they know they will have to keep costs down, sometimes at the expense of good quality care. Worse, there are cases where the NHS should have been paying the fees, but refuses to. In January 2007, Mike Pearce got the nursing home fees returned that had been paid for his highly dependent mother whose condition was so severe she had difficulty doing anything for herself except chewing and swallowing. This is a shocking situation.[14]

These top-up fees remain hidden, which makes those paying for their own care especially vulnerable. Yet local authorities wash their hands of them, providing almost nothing in the way of advice or information.

Poor care

When I was researching this book, I found more examples of really good care than I was expecting, often provided by small organizations, or by charities, even though they sometimes failed to live up to the required room size and standard that our bureaucracies now insist on. But there is no doubt that there is a great deal of second-rate care around. The broadcaster Jenni Murray talked about the experience of losing her parents in this second-rate world:

> *My mother was a civil servant, housewife and mother;*
> *and then, as I struck out on my adult life, she worked for*
> *the local council as the most elegant, most charming and*
> *helpful receptionist she could be. She's still something of*
> *a legend in the local town hall. They lived in the same*
> *small town of Barnsley all their lives, working for mental*
> *health charities in their spare time and running the local*
> *badminton club to give young people somewhere to go.*
> *They – and I – never expected that, as their lives drew to*
> *a close, when the state should have been paying back*
> *something of their law-abiding loyalty, patriotism and*
> *fierce independence, there would be nothing on offer. My*
> *mother ended her life in inadequate care in an*
> *understaffed, commercial nursing home. My father had*
> *excellent care and died in a hospice – a movement*
> *founded not by the government, but begun and sustained*
> *by charity."*[15]

Jenni Murray had no complaints about the kindness of the staff, but the home was understaffed, radiators never got fixed, her mother's hair was never done and lipstick was never put on, and the contrast with the hospice where her father died a few months later was incredible. Care shouldn't be like that.

On the other hand, when the care is bad there are some truly terrible stories, like the ones that came out about the Maypole nursing home in King's Heath, Birmingham, where 28 residents died in one year. These came to light when a resident choked to death, and it transpired that the previous year (2001) only nine deaths had happened. The home was run by two GPs, who were eventually struck off, and the report of the initial inquiry into the home found that – while there was no suggestion that residents were harmed deliberately – some patients were not given 'the appropriate drugs, at the appropriate dosage, at the appropriate times'.[16]

The review highlighted the 'wholly inappropriate' use of deep, reclining 'bucket chairs' and the fear that they may have been used as a method of restraint. Once in them, immobile residents were unable to get out, and officials feared the lack of mobility could have speeded the onset of pneumonia, as well as worsening pressure sores, which are seriously painful.

Residents died of ailments common in older people, such as pneumonia, but officials involved in the review noted 'rapid progress from the onset of illness to death, significantly outside the normal range for bronchopneumonia'. In some cases, there were no records indicating that the person who died had been suffering from bronchopneumonia immediately before death anyway. The General Medical Council frowns upon, but does not forbid, doctors who own nursing homes being the residents' GPs – and signing their death certificates – though it should.

There are related stories all the time – Parkfields Residential Care Home in Butleigh, Somerset, closed within days in 2007 following a 'total lack of co-operation' by the owners of the home.[17] There was Westergate House Care Home in Fontwell, West Sussex, involving a death from septicaemia which may have been the result of a residents' pressure sores.

Pressure sores emerge as a theme time and time again. They can cause enormous pain and distress, as well as infection. The use of bucket chairs, the failure to use pressure aids, the lack of regular turning, and the lack of rubbing of feet or other affected parts, are all contributory factors, and care homes and nursing homes should be asked about the level of training for dealing with pressure sores as a regular part of basic care.

Those bucket seats are pretty horrible by anyone's reckoning. The Maypole nursing home used them in great numbers. In Roger Graef's *Dying for the Truth* film for the BBC in 2006, Hazel Bicknell described being asked to buy a bucket seat for her father in Maypole. It cost £800, and she thought it sounded a caring thing to do. It was never bought because he died only eight days after arriving there. Mrs Bicknell describes her father's body as 'contorted' and believes he had been placed in a bucket seat. The *Independent* commented: 'Bucket seats are something akin to an instrument of torture. They are used as a method of forcible restraint. They look comfy but actually engulf and immobilize the frail, rendering them unable to get up and walk about, or even lean forward and adjust their sitting position. They inflict horrible bedsores and constrict the ability of the chest to expel fluid.'[18]

There are continual stories about accidents with hoists, often when equipment – well designed and excellent when used properly – is used inappropriately, with too few staff or with staff who haven't been trained. There are, on the other hand, stories about deliberate abuse, like the Laurel Bank nursing home in Halifax where Agnes Moore stayed for so-called respite care after her husband died. Whilst she was there, she was badly and painfully lifted, and a sore on her back that she arrived with was so badly treated that she developed septicaemia.

The BBC report into Laurel Bank in Halifax found complaints from a resident that staff had allegedly punched her in the stomach and threatened her by waving scissors in her face, of older residents being verbally abused – staff were allegedly overheard using sexually aggressive language and asking a resident questions about her sex life and her body – of regular understaffing and criminal record checks on new staff not always being made. One care worker who worked at Laurel Bank until October 2003 described how difficult residents or those without relatives were kept in the so-called 'loopy lounge', and an old lady allegedly being slapped with wet flannels.[19]

Often this abuse comes in the form of heavy sedation. Mary Riddell wrote in the *Observer* about the mother of a friend who became mildly confused after breaking her hip in a care home. But on one visit she recognized her daughters and spoke lucidly. They were told that her pills had been stopped while she was given antibiotics. 'Suspicious, they discovered that her normal drug was actually a remedy for schizophrenics that had left her mute, helpless, and tractable as a doll,' wrote Mary Riddell:

> *Staff said that medication would start again. Otherwise*
> *her daughters could take her away. They should see how*
> *they liked it when she wept in the undrugged moments of*
> *terror that her dementia induced. Her family has found*
> *no solution yet. They watch their mother sitting in a chair*
> *all day and staring at nothing, still as a stone apart from*
> *one trembling hand. She is almost 100 now, and caught,*
> *like many, in a pocket of pointless time.*[20]

Care home closures

Closures are accelerating, and they can have devastating consequences. They are, in their way, another form of abuse. Some owners are finding they can get more for their properties, particularly in the south and west of the country, by simply selling them on the open market. Others are finding the regulatory framework, especially around room size, will cost them too much to carry on. Others find they simply can't make enough money from running care and nursing homes, as local authorities drive down what they are willing to pay. Some owners say they would rather go out of business than provide a level of care they themselves would not be happy with. Many local authority homes have been closing as well.

Many older people who live in care or nursing homes – their homes, after all – are complaining bitterly about having to move against their will, with little in the way of options about where to go. But it is hard to fight closures. Campaigners fighting a decision by Staffordshire County Council to axe 22 care homes and nine day centres won a respite in March 2007, after getting an emergency injunction stopping the authority from moving residents.[21] Yvonne Hossacks, a lawyer who specializes in care home closure cases, represented 80 families affected by the Staffordshire decision. She referred to her own experience advising the residents of a care home in Kettering, Northamptonshire, where one home closed in 1998. Within a year of its closure 15 out of 41 former residents had died.

Back in 2001, Niall Dickson – now chief executive of the King's Fund – reported at length for the BBC on the emerging crisis. At that stage, Kent, the country's largest local authority, had lost 22 per cent of its nursing home beds in the previous twelve months, and had no beds at all for dementia patients in some parts of the county.

'It is hard to imagine what it must be like to be 98 years old and to learn that you must leave the care home where you have lived for the past 15 years,' said Dickson. 'You are given just a few weeks to say goodbye to the staff and friends who form the backbone of your life, it is cruel and it is happening every day.'[22]

Ken Mack, 65, who had been fighting the closure of two council-run care homes in Wrexham, delivered a letter to 10 Downing Street to make his case early in 2007 and urged some kind of Bill of Rights for all frail and elderly people. Rose Cottle, 102, famously took to the streets as a retired teacher to demonstrate in Downing Street about the closure of the home she had lived in for 15 years, the Borehamwood Care Village in Hertfordshire. 'How much longer are we going to ignore the mounting death toll among the elderly arising from official parsimony, buck-passing and negligence?' wrote Melanie Phillips in the *Daily Mail*.[23] She was writing about Winifred Humphrey, also 102, who had died just 16 days after being evicted from her state-funded place in the care home she had lived in for nine years, to make room for a fee-paying resident.

Only a few weeks before, Violet Townsend, 88, died from acute stress five days after being moved from her care home in Gloucestershire. The council funding Mrs Townsend refused to pay the extra fees and moved her instead, despite her doctor's warning that the move would kill her. The coroner then refused to let the doctor register the cause of death as acute stress, forcing him to enter it instead as 'old age'.

Phillips argued that the crisis arose from a swindle by the local authorities. Whilst the government had given them a six per cent increase for social service spending, the majority were spending some of this on other things, giving care homes far less money. That was partly true: they had to do something because of central government instructions to put more resources into services for children and vulnerable young people. It is not entirely the fault of the local authorities, though you have to ask why the axe has to fall on the most vulnerable.

In the summer of 2007, the Law Lords got involved in the case of *Johnson v the London Borough of Havering*, about a group of elderly residents in Havering, East London, who feared that their human rights would be compromised if the council went ahead with plans to transfer its care homes to a private-sector provider. The campaigners who wanted to bring the case said the law needed to be changed, or clarified, to prevent elderly couples being separated in care, or care homes closed without the consent of vulnerable residents.

They lost the case. As it stands, though government has recently promised to change it, the law gives residents in independent homes less protection if the owners decide to close it. And while local authorities have a duty to assess anyone who may need a community care service it provides, and a statutory duty to arrange suitable accommodation for anyone they are already funding in the current home, they have no such duty to self-funders. The council may also have some duty to find alternatives for self-funding residents if no one else is available to help, but that appears to be very limited, if it exists at all.

Care workers

Counsel and Care held a series of more than 50 seminars with care home workers, and kept hearing of residents 'being deprived of walking frames and rails placed around their beds to control movement'. They concluded that staff shortages were the biggest cause of the misuse of restraint and called for better training and pay for care home staff.

That is the core problem. When the King's Fund investigated in 2001, they found that between 900,000 and 1.2 million care workers had few qualifications, virtually none relevant, were underpaid, that staff turnover was high and likely to get worse as the workers themselves got older, and that the staff were looking to the retail sector for lighter work with better pay.[24] Traditionally female work, care home care assistants did it because that was all they could get. But given fuller employment and a lack of willingness to accept such low pay for work held in such low esteem, the system was near collapse.

Over the last 30 years or more, we have seen the professionalization of nursing, in particular, where nurses are now university graduates with training that makes them technically very proficient, increasingly research driven, and increasingly advisory to other junior staff or the deliverers of hi-tech intervention. At the same time, they are often unskilled in basic hands-on procedures, because that was not part of their training. Meanwhile, the actual hands-on caring is delivered by care assistants, whose training is often minimal and whose security of tenure, and relationship with the rest of the staff, tends to be poor.

The status of nurses has risen, and the former 'slave labour' demanded of student nurses has, by and large, disappeared. But they no longer provide the discipline and structure to a care home or nursing home, ward or hospital in the way that they used to. The regular job of caring for sick people and vulnerable older people, emptying their bed pans and giving them their meals, turning them and making them comfortable, has been handed 'down' – in the hierarchy – to care assistants. Nurses are just too expensive now to feed patients, make beds and plump up pillows. So the people who are performing the most intimate tasks for the patients, most of whom are old, are the care assistants.

Many of these are truly wonderful people. Many of them are largely untrained. National Vocational Qualifications are increasingly common, and many hospitals, care homes and nursing homes encourage their care assistants to take those exams. But not all of them are willing to pay for the training, or give time off for it. Many of them do not pay more if someone has got the qualification. Yet if employers could provide incentives to get training, and continue up the ladder into nursing, the whole atmosphere might change. Care assistants would be seen as would-be nurses. The role of wiping bottoms, cleaning people up, washing them, feeding them, would not be seen as dirty, skivvy work, but something you do on the way up.

In care homes and nursing homes, what may well be needed is a sense that those providing the care are not short-term employees, doing dirty work for little money and no emotional and 'respect' reward, but people who may go into nursing eventually, or who may choose to remain as care assistants, at the top of that tree, with all its attendant qualifications and respect, because what they actually want to do is look after vulnerable, frail or sick people.

The government set itself the target of half of all care home staff having reached NVQ level 2 by 2005. That never happened. But by 2006 they had decided to set up a registration scheme for all social care workers, from social workers to care home assistants. This will be slow, but it is the right thing to do, even though it is likely to make care staff more expensive, because it might raise their status. However, it doesn't tackle the problem of training. It isn't clear that most care home employers will even pay the registration fees to General Social Care Council for their staff. One poll suggested that only 55 per cent would do so, which is pretty shocking.

It is unlikely that the government's target will be reached by 2010, but their intentions are good, and grants given to care home owners to help them pay for courses and study leave would speed up the process. Meanwhile, the work is hard, often physically back-breaking. It can also often be unrewarding, because patients with Alzheimer's disease, for instance, can be unresponsive or abusive or both at the same time. The shifts are long and often too busy with tasks. Time to sit and talk to residents is limited, and the culture doesn't value it.

This is another core problem. The culture of care homes and care at home regards tenderness, care and a bit of quality time spent with the patients as wasteful. This is by no means universal. Many residents in nursing homes and care homes sing the praises of particular staff, and have clearly developed strong relationships with them. Staff who genuinely enjoy the company of older people, and who have the time to sit with them and hear about their lives, often get great satisfaction from what they are doing. But until these staff are paid better, it will be left to individuals within particular care and nursing homes to behave differently.

Until care assistants have real status, they will not – as a group – tend to give of their best. Until they are trained and recognized, there will always be the risk of abuse from people who may know no better – or, more frightening still, can get no other work. It is still all too easy to walk into a care home, or into an agency, and get work looking after the vulnerable there and then.

This is the heart of the conundrum. Care assistants are appallingly badly treated. We have allowed our most vulnerable older people to be cared for by people to whom we show no respect. We have to do this properly, pay properly, train properly and support properly, the people who do the back-breaking work day after day, without the cost of care becoming prohibitive. Unless we do so, care workers and assistants will be encouraged to provide the most intimate care without a sense of self-worth.

'If we don't value teachers, we insult carers,' wrote Janet Street-Porter.[25] Until we stop doing so, we will get the carers we deserve.

Divided couples

Of all the examples of appalling care I found while I was research-ing this book, alongside even more examples of good care, there was one trend that I found deeply disturbing. This was the separation of married couples by social services to provide for their care needs, something so inconceivable as to be beyond belief – but it happens.

The *Daily Mail* took up the case of the Dunnells, who had been married for six decades. Betty Dunnell, 80, had been put on the wait-ing list for a council-owned flat with round-the-clock care. But her husband Eric, 85, was told by Norfolk County Council that she was too healthy to be eligible and must stay living in their bungalow. 'Every time I think about it I want to burst into tears,' said Mrs Dunnell. 'We've never done anything wrong and now we're being punished.'[26]

This and similar stories reflect the shortage of care home places, as well as a lack of flexibility. They may be based on the worst kind of penny-pinching, but might not always be quite all they seem, as Christopher Manthorp, operations manager for old people's serv-ices in Kent, wrote in the *Guardian* in 2006:

> *These kinds of decisions involve love, money and well-intentioned legislation, the perfect recipe for a complete mess. My 30 years experience in residential care has not exposed me to an overdose of blissful marital happiness. Many people who have spent 65 years in each other's company are sick of the sight of each other; if brought in*

as couples to shared rooms, they will flee promptly to
opposite ends of the building.[27]

These problems are individual and far from simple for any bureau-cracy. But the worst accusation against the old poorhouses was that they divided married couples, and to divide people because of budgets is uncivilized and inhumane.

Pain relief

The other emerging theme is the worrying evidence about the levels of pain that residents in nursing and care homes end up suffering. A recent study for the Patients' Association found that nearly two out of five residents experienced constant pain. In fact, the majority of the 77 people they asked said that no doctor or nurse had ever talked to them about how their pain could be relieved.[28] 'I will cry every night nearly, the pain is so bad,' said one 95-year-old woman they talked to. 'It makes you wish you were dead, you wish you were and you think I wish it would happen soon – the older you get the damn worse it is.' Eight per cent described their pain as excruciating.

In every case, where there were discussions about pain management, they took place between the GP and the nursing staff in the home, rather than with the residents themselves. No one seems to have been asked how they felt about the pain. Indeed, pain-relieving medicines were dispensed as a routine, rather than in response to an individual's pain levels or type of pain. Given that chronic pain is a common problem for older people, which can significantly reduce their quality of life, this is a quite extraordinary finding.

The research found that 90 per cent of those questioned said it limited the activities they could take part in and 38 per cent said it made them feel depressed and miserable. Three quarters of them had experienced the severe pain for over a year, without much in the way of relief – or indeed, much concern amongst staff. Of those who suffered, 57 per cent had never been asked about their pain by care home staff and 85 per cent had never spoken to a doctor or nurse about pain relief.

For some reason, both staff and residents seemed to accept pain as an inevitable consequence of growing old. At least part of the problem lies in the fact that older people get cut off from their GPs and other health providers when they go into a care home, and the level of primary care cover varies hugely from home to home.

Clearly, this evidence was seriously alarming. All the charities responded by saying how disgraceful the situation was, and the Royal College of GPs is working with the Patients' Association and the British Pain Society to produce guidelines on management of persistent pain. But the Department of Health came up with a luke-warm response to a report that was deeply shocking, saying that all nursing homes should provide residents with access to any care they needed from hospitals and community health services, 'according to their individual medical needs'. Well, of course.

But the government did list some of those care needs and it included chiropody, or podiatry as it is described more often these days. Feet are of huge importance to older people. Jackie Morris, a consultant geriatrician, has done magnificent presentations that demonstrate this in her talks about ageing well and frailty.[29] She says that a quarter of people aged over 65 have foot problems requiring podiatry, often just because of the difficulty of cutting their toe-nails because of osteoarthritis of the hips or knees, or other causes such as diabetes.

But because podiatry is rarely free on the NHS these days, the consequences – if people can't afford to go to the podiatrist or have them come to them at home or in their nursing home – are 'foot pain, poor mobility, being housebound, exclusion, and lack of engagement'.

Good care

Some things are changing in ways that prove it is possible to make things work. Some people are becoming live-in carers in return for a nominal rent and no bills, through an organization called Homeshare. Many younger people find the housing market in London really difficult, and this is one way to live somewhere nice, in exchange for some relatively light caring duties. 'We're really happy here,' Nick Shepley told the *Guardian* in 2007.[30] 'I've learned a new perspective. Seeing two people deal with older age so gracefully and accept us into their home is a unique experience – it's a shame it doesn't happen more.'

Homeshare was originally the brainchild of Nan Maitland, who recognized that many older people have spare space, and even a second bathroom. They may be property rich and not want to move, but they are often cash poor. This means giving space to young people who want a home in exchange for light care, and should be a godsend for both sides.

It certainly worked for my mother, who had 'homesharers' for the last five years of her life. One of the homesharers even got married from my mother's flat. It deals with loneliness and isolation, helps young people – often foreign students – get accommodation, and it leads to considerable enrichment on both sides. But still only a minority of people do this.

In Germany, bizarrely, they are using prostitutes as care workers, taking them off the streets in the state of North Rhine Westphalia, paid for by the state.[31] The project is based on the idea that prostitutes are good at dealing with people, have no fear of physical contact and make excellent carers of the elderly. Officials say that they are often better at the job than trainee nurses.

These examples all show that we don't necessarily need to hurtle towards the dystopia where we seem to be heading, but they are little more than indications that another future is possible.

Food

As chairman of a big NHS trust in central London in the mid-1990s, I was only too well aware of the likes and dislikes of many of the patients on our longer-stay 'care of the elderly' wards. Steamed pudding was a great favourite, and some of the older women, with bird-like frames, would lap up huge portions as though their lives depended on it – and, in a way, they did. Steamed pudding is easy to eat, soft, sweet, nourishing, and very familiar. It takes relatively little agility with cutlery for frail older people to manage it, and washed down with plenty of custard, made with full cream milk, it probably provided most of the calories they needed for the day.

At that stage, on those wards, we still had our own cooks preparing the food – wonderful men and women who would come in at 3 a.m. on Christmas morning to get the turkeys into the ovens ready for a slap-up meal, and who also knew how important it was to cut things up into small pieces. More recently, food in hospitals has been of varying quality, often pre-frozen and brought in ready to be thawed and cooked. Jay Rayner described one hospital meal as: 'Thick salty soup with the texture of wallpaper paste; a pie crust, hiding a serving of mechanically recovered "meat" and dry mash.'[32] The Department of Health has very quietly disbanded Loyd Grossman's food panel dedicated to improving food in hospitals, even though they know there is a problem about malnutrition for older people on leaving hospital and, all too often, going into hospital as well. The Department of Health also knew that there were widespread complaints more generally: up 64 per cent between 2001 and 2006 (the *Daily Mail* also reveals that £162 million worth of hospital food has been thrown away in the last five years).

'Pretty grim, isn't it? I've lost a stone, can't believe that,' said Bert Geddes, indicating his hospital meal, because the hospital can't match his vegetarian diet.[33] Yet we know older people rate food as a key part of successful ageing. Bert's regime is not that unusual. It might be argued that hospitals, and other institutions such as care homes, just have to catch up with the population.

But that is to jump ahead to details of healthcare in the next chapter. The problem of food is even sharper in care, where the Commission for Social Care and Inspection has urged care homes to involve older people in decisions about meals and their presentation. One correspondent of mine, Geoff Gilbert from Humberstones in the West Country, a valuer for companies involved in the care home sector, told me that he was often shocked at the quality and quantity of food provided in care homes. He mentioned one home where there was only a choice of two possible breakfast cereals, because the group of care homes bought them in bulk. This is not any old home either but among the most upmarket homes in the West Country. He argued that the cost of food provided in many care homes was at £2.50–£3 a day, around £1,000 a year, probably less than the cost of incontinence pads for the same period. Yet these are homes charging upwards of £450 a week, up to £25,000 a year – or more for nursing homes – with food being a minute proportion of the costs incurred by care providers. I was talking about food at a conference recently for the care home industry, and several of the attendees came up to me afterwards and said how ashamed they were about the row upon row of cook-chill and freezer cabinets and the lack of any fresh food at all.

Fran Abrams went undercover to investigate food in care homes in 2006.[34] At one home in Streatham, in South London, she stood in the dining room with several older residents already seated at tables, and the care manager looked rather surprised at the questions Abrams was asking. 'Were the vegetables freshly cooked, I wanted to know? No, she said. They sometimes came out of the freezer. And the soup that was served up every single evening for supper? Was it home-made? No, she said. It came out of a packet. The bread, it transpired, was usually white and pre-sliced.' With the possibility that four out of every ten residents in care homes being malnourished, this is serious stuff.

The Malnutrition Advisory Group, an expert group of doctors and other health experts, has warned that one in seven people over the age of 65 in the UK is malnourished, or at severe risk of malnutrition. Apparently, this is most pronounced in the North West, where one in five of the over-65s is undernourished. But despite a North–South divide in the case of general malnutrition, when it comes to nursing homes, where around one in four older people will spend their last days, malnutrition rates are more generally one in five. Up to 10 per cent of nursing home residents lose five per cent of their body weight within a month of admission, and 10 per cent of their body weight within six months.

Given that older people themselves describe eating well, and enjoying their food, as an important part of ageing well, the figures for malnutrition are shocking and dramatic. As one probes deeper, the reasons are complicated. Some people are too frail to get to the shops, and get meals delivered or ready prepared, less attractive meals than they are used to. Others have difficulty preparing meals and live on biscuits and chocolate, with the occasional treat of a piece of cheese, as one old lady told me. Some are simply ill, and cannot face their food, rendering them weaker and slower to recover. They then eat the various food supplement drinks, because they are easier, although no one I have ever met describes themselves as having a taste for them.

Yet malnutrition leads to a whole variety of responses, all of which are destructive of the will to live and a sense of well-being: immune responses are impaired, leading to greater susceptibility to infection, muscle strength diminishes and fatigue ensues. Breathing can become more difficult; thermo-regulation becomes impaired, with the person feeling the cold to a dramatic extent, wounds heal badly, and the person becomes apathetic, often depressed, and self-neglectful, as well as having a poor libido. In other words, they begin to behave as if they don't think it is worth carrying on living, when in fact it is the malnutrition that is making them feel like that and not their calendar age at all.

Even at home, where people are likely to get meals on wheels, more than a quarter of patients receiving district nursing care are thought to be malnourished.[35] Meanwhile, of those who are home-bound, the figure varies hugely, and is anything between 44 and 55 per cent of housebound older adults.[36] These are huge figures, and therefore the issue of meals provision at home ought to be taken very seriously. But there are problems here too.

In practice, there is considerable local variation in how meals are provided and delivered, although there is an increasing trend towards the delivery of frozen meals for those capable of using them. The WRVS has been, and continues to be, a major player in the provision and delivery of meals, and other voluntary sector providers are still involved. But the service is increasingly outsourced to private companies.

In February 2006, Chorley MP Lindsay Hoyle paid tribute to the WRVS in a House of Commons debate:

> *I was dragged in to help on a snowy day when people were struggling to deliver meals and I saw that even those who were not taking a meal enjoyed the visit. The fact that people took time out to have a few words with them mattered so much. I have witnessed at first hand the value of such contact. If someone wants their chair pulled up to the table, the person delivering the meal can do that for them and help in many other ways ... I wonder how on earth the county council has got itself to the point that it has with the proposal that we are discussing. If we consider what the WRVS does, we see that the issue should not be all about financial savings. In fact, we should be asking the WRVS how it does such a good job and how we can enhance the service. Instead, we hear people say, 'There is an alternative. We will employ a company to deliver a freezer and people can have seven meals.'[37]*

'Who will go round and check that things are okay?' asked Lindsay Hoyle. 'How much will it cost to check on pensioners and the vulnerable? Will that mean more social workers and more home visits? What if someone does not cook a meal properly? What will be the cost of that? We all know what the consequences will be. All the value that people get from a hot meal could disappear and their nutrition could be affected. There will be a reduction in social contact, which could lead to a deterioration in people's well-being and a subsequent reduction in healthiness.'

It is easy to sympathize, but the arguments are not absolutely clear. For a start, old-style hot meals were not, and are not, universally popular and many customers felt that a no-choice menu was unacceptable. The delivery of hot meals inevitably means that not everyone can receive a meal at the same time. This often results in a two-hour delivery slot, and some people may receive their lunch soon after 11.30 a.m., whilst others may not get their lunch until almost 2 p.m. It could be argued that delivering a daily meal might even deter older people from going out if they are able to do so. If they do go out – even to a hospital appointment – they may miss their meal entirely. Frozen meals offer more choice and more flexibility, although without the daily social contact of the delivery person.

Even so, WRVS is right when it says that 'levels of loneliness will increase'.[38] There is little doubt that many older people look forward to and rely on the brief contact they get from the volunteers or paid workers who deliver their meals. A minimal level of additional help, such as putting the meal on the plate, is undoubtedly welcomed by many of the most disabled. But maybe we should be asking why older people in particular, or the general public of all ages, feel it is acceptable to settle for so little in the way of contact, or indeed of choice of food? What sort of society is it that relies on a two-minute daily visit to check on someone's well-being and provide social contact? And are meals on wheels the way to provide contact anyway? Is it that meals on wheels are seen as a necessary delivery, meaning that older people do not need to think they are being 'checked up on' if the WRVS lady just pops in with a meal and says hello?

While home-delivered meals are usually most appropriate for those who are not particularly mobile, there is clearly scope to improve access to lunch clubs and other forms of sociable dining. Improved and accessible transport is a key to this. A more imaginative approach could also have huge benefits. One scheme in Herefordshire is an example of this with an inter-generational lunch club which encourages older people to join the children in St Mary's Primary School for lunch.

In fact, there is a worrying lack of a link between meals on wheels as a concept and other forms of meals provision. In rural Ireland, where services can be very patchy, there are some examples of meals being cooked by local women and brought to the older person or people concerned, where the person who prepared the meal sits down to eat it with them, sometimes accompanied by small children.

This has the added advantage of allowing older people to have a considerable say about what they get to eat. It also encourages a more 'family' feel to mealtimes, and a longer conversation by far. It is undoubtedly expensive and, from what I could gather, largely paid for by the people concerned, rather than being provided as a regular service by the local authority. Even so, a scheme like that would have considerable attraction for older people who are not at all badly off financially, but are lonely and see few children. It would turn a lonely exercise in shovelling fuel into one's mouth into a serious time of social engagement. The increasing move towards direct payments to service users, often unpopular with social services departments, should eventually extend choice for how older people get their meals, if they can't make their own. If and when it does, I hope it will include a choice of schemes like that.

Dignity in care

One of the persistent themes, particularly in this chapter, is the way that older people are not given the dignity they deserve by those who are paid to look after them. This is really a matter of treating the recipients of care as equals. It isn't very hard to understand this, but, as care givers, people seem to find it hard to do. So it was especially heart-warming to find two gerontologists from Trinity College, Dublin, arguing hard for a different language to be used in care.

Marianne Falconer and Desmond O'Neill rejected the word 'elderly' as pejorative in any other context, obscuring the wisdom, experience, enhanced creativity, strategic skills and maturity that are often overlooked in an ageist society.[39] It also obscures the great variability between individuals, since older populations are more complex and heterogeneous than younger cohorts. It was wonderful to read them questioning whether we would regard the great and late works of Verdi and Matisse as works of 'older' artists.

They are not alone. There are increasing numbers of campaigns to provide dignity in care, whatever the setting. The government started its own such campaign in November 2006, while the *Daily Mail* has been running its enormously effective and influential Dignity in Care Campaign, and has probably pushed government more than the older people's charities ever could.

Sometimes this means learning from models in other countries. Daelhoven in the Netherlands has a 120-bed home, split off into six-bed wings for people with dementia. It is well designed and has a café bar where local residents can go for a drink or to eat, because it serves good food. That in itself is a counter to the isolation experienced by residents in all too many care and nursing homes. It also has a large paved central courtyard area, gardens and communal space. Even the most disabled residents help with preparing for and clearing up after meals, which provides a structure to the day and some level of normal activity.

Sometimes it means simple attention to better food, like the Anchor Trust's Dining with Dignity programme. This has many aspects to it, including making food look attractive. Staff are also encouraged to sit with residents and to encourage them to eat, rather than feeding them, if possible, and they practise feeding each other, so they know what it feels like, which is essential if food is not to be pushed into older people's mouths too fast in order to 'get it over with' – which, of course, leads to indigestion, problems with swallowing, and a failure to enjoy one of life's last pleasures.

There is also a campaign being run by the English Community Care Association (ECCA) to get drinking water easily available for care home residents.[40] Their survey found that only a third of homes had water in all communal rooms, and a quarter only made drinking water available when requested. As many as 15 per cent only made it available at meal times.

Sometimes it is about activity, like the project by occupational therapists in Camden in London to train care home staff to create tailor-made activities for people with dementia. Jennifer Wenborn, the therapist concerned, teaches care staff how to record people's life stories and to use the information to introduce daily activities that can improve the quality of their care.[41] This could include simple changes such as making sure the patient's preferred newspaper is available, or that their favourite aromatherapy oil is used at bath time, or having the radio station which is preferred by the residents on, rather than the one the staff prefer. 'People still think that OT is all about organized activity sessions that happen once a week when somebody comes into the home,' she says. 'I am trying to instil the idea that activities are much broader and should be integrated into the day-to-day working of the care staff.'

Some of the best care is still found in dedicated homes for trades or professions, or for specific faith groups. There are still homes run by the Journalists' Charity and the Musicians' Benevolent Fund, among others. Many of these bodies have sold up. The Teacher Support Network has sold off all its homes, though the Teachers' Housing Association runs seven sheltered housing schemes. But there are still a number of them hanging on, like BEN, the occupational fund for people in the motor and related industries.

The shared backgrounds of residents can make life more sociable and these homes may be better able to provide appropriate tailor-made activities. Also vital is the level of interest in the quality of care and general atmosphere shown by younger members of that trade or faith. The group concerned takes 'ownership' of the nursing or care home concerned and, though this isn't always the case, it often leads to a better quality of care and an atmosphere of greater openness, with people from that faith group or trade 'popping in' for a short chat or visit, just to see how things are getting on.

This openness and sense of 'moral ownership' ought to be encouraged, even in very different settings, so that local communities feel a sense of ownership for 'their' care home or nursing home. 'Care establishments, including care homes, can be the hub of the community and schools, amateur dramatic societies and other amenities should be encouraged to interact with them,' says Martin Green of ECCA. 'The business of caring needs to be acknowledged as a profession and supported appropriately in order for older people to receive the high quality care that they require.'[42]

When care homes work well, there tend to be a number of similar themes, including person-centred care and listening to people, maintaining a sense of identity, meaningful activities, a level of participation, a positive social environment, consistent staff assignment, involving people from the local community, enabling residents to contribute to care home life and the local community, enabling residents to be themselves – deciding how to dress, having control over their personal space, a balance between secure storage of personal possessions and enabling residents to use them whenever they want, a recognition of ethnic or cultural needs and spiritual needs, offering couples space for intimacy and privacy, and good care at the end of life.

Take Alfred Hudson, for example. He spent 21 months in a nursing home before going into sheltered accommodation at the age of 83. His first nursing home was less than satisfactory: they forgot to order new pain patches and the painkiller wasn't given to him whenever he asked. But the second was a new family-run home which asked him straight away to help plan his future care and activities:

> I become a member of an advisory group which met to
> explore ways in which life could be improved for
> everyone in the home. It comprised management, staff,
> residents and family. Because standards were already
> high it was difficult to make suggestions, but, jointly, we
> were able to fine-tune some aspects of the system ... I also
> appreciated chats with the nurses and the carers. They
> always had a smile and made me feel as if I was
> important ... I do miss everyone in the nursing home who
> helped me to live such a full life. If necessary, I would be
> more than happy to go back.[43]

'Good small homes are intimate, with a family feel,' wrote Christopher Manthorp in 2006. 'Struggling for money means décor can have a slightly homemade feel but many residents prefer that to the clinical hotel like atmosphere of the more expensive establishments.'[44] Small homes can be claustrophobic, and they are financially much more precarious, so that they are more likely to go out of business. But Manthorp argues that government makes it impossible for small homes through 'fee structures which make a home with anything much less than 30 beds more a vocational hobby than a business'. He wants to combine the virtues of small homes with the strengths of larger establishments.

Call to arms

One of the worst cases I read while I was researching this book was about an older person who was allegedly force-fed talcum powder by her paid carers.[45] Lucy Neal, 89, had been given the powder by care workers at her home in Handsworth, Birmingham. Although the carers who worked for the Welcome Care Agency were cleared of assault in February 2004, the agency admitted negligence in a civil action. It then had its approval removed and its contracts with Birmingham Social Services cancelled, and it subsequently closed down. The incident had been recorded on a video camera set up by Mrs Neal's son, after he became concerned for his mother who had a range of physical and cognitive disorders.

This is an extreme case, and it is hard to blacklist care workers. Some of those blacklisted have successfully complained that the list breaches their human rights. But Help the Aged's Elder Abuse campaign makes it clear that abuse takes a variety of different forms, with about 500,000 older people being abused at any one time in the UK, and many of the abusers are related to the person they are abusing.[46] Two thirds of abuse is committed at home, by someone in a position of trust, and often by more than one person in collusion. So care homes, nursing homes and hospitals are by no means the worst offenders.

Help the Aged says that officials should give abuse of older people the same priority that is given to child abuse, especially when over half the theft and fraud against older people is committed by their own children. Like the case of Brooke Astor, 104, who died in August 2007, who was allegedly mistreated by her only son and bled of money by him – he was in his eighties – and made to sleep on a urine-stained sofa and generally given a rough time.[47]

Puzzling over this and similar cases, the columnist Alexander Chancellor asked how children can be so callous, and answerd the question himself by saying that the parents are 'sitting ducks'. 'It seems incredible that they should allow greed to override their natural affection for, and duty of care towards, the men and women who brought them into the world and nurtured them through childhood,' he wrote. 'They may justify it in their minds by deciding their parents are gaga and need protection from squandering their assets or leaving everything to cats' homes. But it is odd and depressing all the same. Maybe they just resent having been born.'

Another and less charitable explanation may be they are just amazingly, unbelievably greedy and think their parents should get on with it and die, so that they – the children – can have their 'rightful' assets.

Whatever the reasons, the truth is that elder abuse is either increasing substantially, or being reported far more. Ireland has a system of elder abuse officers around the country, and intends to have one in every county to work with public health nurses, doctors, social workers, in care homes and in conjunction with police and legal services, something that might also help in the UK.

There were reports in Italy in 2005 that 10–20 per cent of those over 70 on Italian hospital wards who could have been discharged for the Christmas season stayed there throughout, because relatives made excuses to keep them in care. In France, too, there were scandals about French old people dying of dehydration in a heat wave during summer 2004, when families were away, as were the staff in many hospitals and clinics. The NHS prided itself – despite regular scandals about hospital-acquired infections – that at least that would not happen in Britain. We had a national system, with decisions being made about which hospitals would be on 'take' over busy Bank Holiday periods, with rostering and planning in each institution, which made such a scenario impossible.

Actually, of course, older people are abandoned in the UK over the summer too – just not quite so comprehensively, because families stagger their holiday dates more than in France.

There may be nothing much the manifesto can specify about sheer greed, though clearly we need to take elder abuse more seriously. These things are able to take place partly because so much of what happens to older people in our society happens in a dim light, away from the media or public attention. If we can make the care of older people more open, and treat those we pay to do it rather better – if we can stop this slide towards considering age as shameful in itself – then there will be less abuse.

But good paid care is crucial to so much else. If we can organize the right kind of care for people at home, then they will grasp the opportunity to stay independent. If we can care for people in nursing homes effectively, the chances are they will get better and go home again. All that depends on us tackling the problem of society's contempt, not just for older people, but for those who care for them. **The government, local authorities and employers need to hammer out and fund a plan to make being a care assistant into a real profession – honourable, well-trained, better paid and giving the chance to rise up into nursing.**

Of all the changes we need to make to the way care is delivered, that is the one that is most far-reaching. But it also needs to be accompanied by changes in the way agency and local authority care staff are employed. The miserable reduction of care workers into harried, clock-watching automatons – with no time for human interaction – is one of the most damaging recent shifts, and is corroding the quality of care all the time. Part of the problem is that they are employed by large agencies, covering very wide areas, treated so badly that staff turnover is appalling.

One solution is that **care workers should form many more local co-operatives, where they also own the business,** and can – simply because they are more local – save a great deal of time which they used to spend just driving around. That shift should also do a great deal to humanize care. There is no reason, for example, when they are self-employed and more local – though also still registered – why they could not, for example, take their children with them: the older people would often enjoy it.

The manifesto also needs to include demands to:

- **Fund an increase in care with a small hypothecated inheritance tax.** That would cost the average estate of £80,000 only £2,000, but it would make an enormous difference to the kind of care that we can provide. It would not mean, normally, that people would have to sell their homes. Unless something along these lines is organized, the chances are that funded care may disappear completely for everyone except those who are most in need, or become so technocratic and inhumane as to be impossible for loving children to allow their parents to be exposed to.

- **Negotiate a new settlement between older people and the state so that people will be expected to pay for two years of care, but the state will pay the rest.** This would hand some of the responsibility for paying for long-term care back on to people, which is right. But it would then end means testing and the unfairness and peculiar differences in what is available around the country, and it would make better care possible again. It is estimated that £5.9 billion is spent every year by private individuals on personal social care for older people alone.[48] They must know what they are entitled to and, if they have to pay for themselves, receive an assurance they will get a fair deal – otherwise those costs will fall increasingly on the state.

- **Make sure that the regulator, whoever it is in future, is involved in raising the status of care work by insisting on proper training.** We desperately need to raise the status of care workers, both in their own eyes and in the eyes of the public, and to regard what they do as the honourable, vital and difficult work that it is.

- **Force local authorities to take responsibility for people paying for their own care home places in their area.** The Office of Fair Trading said that people need easier access to information when choosing a care home and more support once in a home. They also need to make sure that the costs and contract terms are fair and transparent. Their recommendation was that the government should set up a central information point for clear information about care for older people, but local authorities also need to take responsibility for all older people in their area – and see that they are fairly treated, get the information they need, and can find a suitable care home place.

- **Double the expenses that care home residents are allowed to keep from their pension.** That would make an enormous difference to them, and allow them to take more responsibility for their own care by paying, for example, for podiatry and other care they need which either isn't available on the NHS or has waiting lists so long that it might as well not be.

- **Organize a massive expansion of mutual care.** Older people are a vital under-used resource, providing different kinds of support for neighbours – perhaps, as in time banks, in return for the right to help for themselves when necessary. Their status inside care homes is higher in the places where they are asked for help managing the day-to-day life of the home. And their involvement as local outsiders in their nearest care home would do more than almost anything else to open them up to the light of day.

- **Change local funding arrangements to encourage small, family-run care homes.** At the moment, these are discouraged by the way payments are made. The result is that homes are increasingly large, less human places, where relationships are even more difficult to build with staff and where rules are even more inflexible. Humane, homely care homes tend to be smaller, and it is insane that we are allowing them to close in such large numbers.

- **Give older people a choice of what to eat at home, how it is delivered and who they will eat with.** Meals on wheels are a vital service, delivered by dedicated volunteers, but they are not a substitute for proper company, especially if those who get their meals delivered have to stay in rather than miss their lunch.

Chapter 8

Don't treat me like I'm not worth repairing

Community beds and hospitals

As Sir Norman Wisdom sits alone in his spartan room in an anonymous nursing home in the Isle of Man, he must wonder how it has come to this. The floor is covered in lino, the hospital-style bed uncomfortably hard. His furniture consists of two plastic chairs, a plastic wardrobe and a plastic chest of drawers. There are few mementoes, rarely any visitors, and little to break up the monotony of his days.

Mail on Sunday, 11 August 2007, revealing that Sir Norman Wisdom's family won't let his friends see him in his confused state

The diarrhoea was unrelenting, but there were just not enough nurses to cope. In the end they gave up trying to get her to the toilet and she was left lying in her own mess. She died feeling embarrassed and humiliated. She did not want her family to visit because the room smelled constantly. I'm so angry about the way my mother was treated, but also fearful for my family and other people who may be admitted to hospital. Something has to be done to stop this.

Ann Cunningham, *Daily Mail*, **10 October 2006, describing the last days of her mother, who contracted two superbugs in hospital and was left to die in her own excrement by harassed hospital staff**

When I was a student in the 1970s, I used to volunteer in a mental hospital near Cambridge, working on what was then a psycho-geriatric ward. One of our jobs was to go round in the mornings with a bucket of false teeth. Everybody's false teeth were put overnight into a huge bucket of sterodent, and we went round in the morning trying to fit the false teeth to the people. They weren't labelled and people could rarely remember who they were, let alone recognize their own teeth. We tried really hard to get it right, but I am sure we very often got it wrong. I was appalled then – and even more appalled now – that we thought it could possibly have been acceptable for people not to have their own cup with their own teeth by their bed on the locker. It was a real objectifying of old people, and the first time I had seen it. It didn't matter to those in authority that their patients couldn't eat properly because their false teeth didn't fit.

It would matter now, so – to that extent at least – things have got better in healthcare. Our treatment of people with mental illness then was pretty bad in hospital, and our treatment of older people with mental problems was truly atrocious. But in some ways, we treated older people without Alzheimer's – which is what those patients without teeth probably had – rather better then than we do now. Because, over the past fifteen years, we have arrived somewhere which is just as bad – and in some ways worse: a terrible attitude at the heart of the administration of the NHS that older people are worth less than the rest of us.

It is that institutional attitude, behind the allocation of scarce resources – rather than the work of a handful of perverse individuals – which has delivered us into the current health crisis, where we have seen older people left to die in their own excrement on Dickensian hospital wards, condemned as 'bed blockers' for being there – when the community hospitals they ought to have been in have been closed down – and denied specialist care and specialist referrals. Just because they are older.

Much of the preceding chapters has been about care, and particularly nursing and social care, help with everyday tasks and help when confused. But older people get ill in the ordinary way as well. Muriel Gillick is a professor at Harvard Medical School and her excellent book *The Denial of Ageing* revealed how we change our attitudes as people get older – both the individuals themselves and their healthcare professionals.[1] Her work is particularly important for this debate in the UK, because there is now overwhelming evidence of discrimination in healthcare against older people. She points out that the situation in the USA is the other way around. Older people are over-treated there, at least until they become very old indeed, whilst the UK experience is that older people – not the very old – don't usually get access to care that would be made available as standard to anyone in their forties or fifties.

Gillick accuses the American system of failing to do sensible, life-enhancing things, while constantly displaying a passionate belief in hi-tech diagnosis and cure. Over the very same period, we had a series of scandals in the UK about how older people were treated within NHS hospitals, including heated rows over the allegation that some six out of ten older people leave hospital malnourished and dehydrated. The publicity was so bad that, in April 2006, the UK government announced yet another measure to help give old people back their dignity on wards: 'dignity nurses' were to be appointed in each hospital, to make sure that older patients are treated with dignity – as if it were possible for one nurse in each hospital to achieve that. The idea has since been scrapped.

Just before that announcement, the *British Medical Journal* published a review of whether people were being allowed to die at home – and here the problems of the UK and USA are similar, though for different reasons.[2] Despite people overwhelmingly saying that they would prefer to die at home, the UK proportion of home deaths for patients with cancer is actually falling, from 27 per cent in 1994 to 22 per cent in 2003.

In the USA, there are different reasons for this. To get their Medicare hospice programme benefit, people have to opt for no intensive intervention at all. American doctors often regard patients as 'theirs', which can make them reluctant to pass patients on to hospice teams, even when further treatment might well be futile or cruel. Gillick suggests that we are reluctant to accept that being in our 80s and 90s is really old, given advancing life expectancy, as the average older person from Florida often sees more than one doctor a week.[3] These are the wrong things being done for the wrong people – at their request – because they fear death or believe they are immortal. Gillick says that centenarians can also teach us about dying because they tend to stay healthy until they suddenly collapse completely, because they are not subjected to the intensive care of those a decade or so younger.

Americans don't treat the centenarians aggressively because they believe that they are truly old, unlike younger 'old people' who are being over-treated. But in the UK, many people in their seventies and eighties are having difficulty being treated adequately at all. Not only that, but a survey conducted for *Doctor* magazine suggests that one in three doctors thinks old people simply should not be given access to various kinds of surgery if it isn't going to do them good for long.[4] Although the chairman of the BMA's ethics committee, Dr Tony Calland, described it as outrageous to limit care on age grounds, and Age Concern said that the doctors' views were disgraceful, it is clear that this is a growing view. That is the pernicious influence of those Quality Adjusted Life Years, the so-called QALYs, which provide a basis for 'experts' to make decisions on the grounds that they know what is best for us statistically.

Rationing and ageism

Evidence for this discrimination is in Help the Aged's recent report *Too Old,* by their Research on Age Discrimination Project, which found that 40 per cent of people believed that health professionals see older people as a nuisance, and 27 per cent of people aged over 65 say that older people receive worse healthcare than younger people.[5] Any manifesto for old age has to tackle this: we need equality in treatment, equality in the seriousness with which treatment is chosen and given, and equality in the autonomy and value as a person with which all patients are treated.

It is true that age limits were traditionally used to ration services and access to treatment. There was widespread acceptance of that. My father certainly thought, at the end of his life, that he had

had 'a fair innings', and had received his 'fair share' of healthcare. Kidney dialysis was not routinely prescribed for the over-65s well into the 1980s, and geriatric provision was often very poor in the early days of the NHS. The old 'back wards' in psychiatric hospitals were reserved for older patients with dementia, and often much neglected. We imagine somehow that the days of such explicit discrimination are over. Far from it.

Take screening services, for instance. Breast cancer screening has been provided every three years for all women over 50 in the United Kingdom since 1988. But once a woman reaches her 70th birthday, she no longer gets a routine letter inviting her to come in for screening. Women over 70 can make their own appointments, but for some reason – it is unclear why, unless there is a value judgement about their worth – they don't get the automatic letter of invitation.

There is a leaflet provided, produced in association with Age Concern, called 'Over 70? You are still entitled to breast screening'. This explains, very properly, that the risk of breast cancer increases with age, and that it is important that women should continue to be screened every three years. But it does not say why they are not invited routinely. The Advisory Committee on Breast Cancer Screening acknowledges that there is 'a benefit to women who wish to continue being screened after 70'. They say women need to be in good health and have a life expectancy of at least about ten years, and attendance levels fall as people get older, which is why they stop inviting people after the age of 70. Yet one reason attendance falls with age is probably because they are just not invited, and forget to make an appointment for themselves. There is also something odd about excluding the women in precisely the age group where the risk increases.

Of course it is right that people should take responsibility for themselves, and the argument about forgetting is not a very good one if we really believe self-care is important. But the problem is not really about 'forgetting'. For some women, thinking about breast cancer – particularly if they had a mother or sister who had it – is just too painful. Unless the notification for their screening comes, it stays out of sight and out of mind. Women are scared of breast cancer, and some – by no means all – would just avoid screening if it were not offered automatically.

But there is a more worrying point here, which is explained in full in the *Too Old* report.[6] The aim of breast screening is to reduce premature deaths, and statistics suggest that it has been successful in doing this since the programme began in 1988. The idea that someone who may not live more than ten years isn't worth saving is fundamentally ageist. In any case, women's life expectancy is getting longer, along with the entire population's changing life expectancy. A woman of 70 can very reasonably expect to live to 85 or 90 – surely that life must be worth saving, and any argument otherwise has an ageist tinge.

The same applies to cholesterol testing. One of the *Too Old* report's diarists went into a pharmacist to get a cholesterol test and was told it was only for people between 55 and 70. The diarist asked why that was, and was told it was the rule – the government said so. In fact, the pharmacist relented, but people who don't push for the test simply wouldn't get it.

Why is this? Lowering cholesterol in older people extends their lives, but it also arguably improves their quality of life, and it might well prevent them having precisely the kind of stroke or heart attack that would make them very dependent on expensive health and social care services. So there is a good economic argument for testing older people's cholesterol levels. The only explanation for the limit of 70 is that it is deliberately ageist – the life of a person over 70 is worth less, apparently, and it doesn't matter if they have some disabling stroke because they are 'not productive'.

There are many other examples, but one that most disturbed me was reading something from a social worker who had also contributed to the *Too Old* report. This is what she said:

> *I was working in a community mental health team for older people when I was asked to assess a gentleman (in his 70s) who had taken to his bed because of severe depression. The GP commented that there was nothing that could be done as 'his time had come'. I arranged for the gentleman to see a psychiatrist who recommended an admission to a psychiatric hospital. Three weeks later the gentleman returned to the community and was able to take up all activities of daily living.*[7]

There are many accounts of people in their seventies and eighties who become depressed after surgery – for instance for a hip replacement – whose depression is left undiagnosed, and where medical and nursing staff just explain their mental state by saying it is the effect of the trauma of the surgery or the effect of the anaesthetic. These are definitely signs of discrimination. Younger people found to be depressed after surgery would be seen by a psychiatrist and their depression taken seriously. There is absolutely no reason in the world why the same shouldn't be true of older people.

Stroke services are one of the clearest examples of discrimination. Access to specialized stroke services is considerably worse for older people than for younger: 71 per cent of patients under 65 are scanned within 24 hours compared with only half of those over 85.[8] Older patients are less likely than younger ones to get some kind of secondary prevention and some aspects of rehabilitation. Brain imaging is performed less often for the over-85s than for younger patients. They are also less likely to be treated in a specialized stroke unit than younger people, and the evidence is clear that standards are consistently better for patients of all ages managed in specialized stroke units than in general wards.

The other worrying feature of health services is in accident and emergency.[9] Those who answered the Help the Aged survey thought they waited longer than younger people before being seen. It is true that A&E staff often believe that 'she's just an old lady and she can wait', that they often forget to give food, drinks and even regular drugs to people waiting, and that they are often seen as less important than younger people. There is no strong sense in the *Too Old* report that this is deliberate, just a very strong feeling that discrimination happens, regularly and observably.

There is the same feeling about the treatment of quite ordinary diseases. A 2007 study found that 46 per cent of GPs and 48 per cent of cardiologists treated patients differently according to their age.[10] Older people were less likely to be prescribed statins, given a cholesterol test, referred to a cardiologist, given an exercise tolerance test, angiography or revascularization. Those doctors who were influenced by age were on average five years older than those who were not. Some of them argued it was right to discriminate, but others were less sure. There is also evidence of discrimination in the exclusion of older people from drug trials for no very good reason.

One thing these studies failed to pick up was how difficult older people often find it to go to a hospital for an appointment. As they become frailer, and find walking long distances harder, they prefer to drive themselves. Most hospitals have too little parking, and it is also often very expensive – understandably, as it is one way for the hospital to make a bit of money. While I was writing this book, I had many letters and messages from people worried about the costs and availability of parking for older people, especially when bus services are often inadequate, and the parking systems are often confusing, expensive and difficult to read.

'I ... noticed how difficult the elderly and disabled patients were finding it to use the new parking machines,' one correspondent wrote to me. 'You have to know your full registration number, the instructions are in small letters and most have to bend almost double to read what to do ... all this and it was pouring with rain to boot that day.'

We will look at dementia in more general terms, but it also provides clear evidence of discrimination. The *British Medical Journal* review devoted a great deal of attention to dementia, arguing that separating NHS medical specialties from psychiatry gets in the way of providing effective, humane and responsive services:

> *Many of these patients present with acute medical problems, particularly delirium, and may be mismanaged. In addition, they are often treated insensitively in mixed sex accommodation and by staff who do not fully understand or know how to plan and organize appropriate care for long term conditions. Half of the patients with moderately severe dementia who enter hospital with acute illnesses such as a chest infection die within six months of admission and fail to receive appropriate palliative or end of life care.*[11]

That, in itself, is a terrible indictment of the way NHS services discriminate against older people: if you are unlucky enough to go into hospital with a chest infection, and you also have dementia, you have a 50:50 chance of dying some months later without proper pain relief.

Bed blockers and re-admissions

There is even stronger evidence that older people are sent back from hospital too soon, putting their lives at risk. A report from Help the Aged called *Spotlight on Older People* shows that more older people than ever have to go back to hospital as emergency cases because they have been discharged from hospital too early.[12] In 2006–7, 147,257 patients over the age of 75 had to be sent back to hospital as emergency cases within 28 days, 33,673 more than two years before, a rise of almost one third.

Some argue that the waiting time targets the government has imposed put pressure on hospitals to discharge patients before they are ready, in order to free up beds. This would explain, to some extent, the appalling use of the term 'bed blockers' to describe older people in beds in NHS acute hospitals who have nowhere else to go. But things may be more complicated. Stringent financial measures over 2006–7 meant that NHS trusts have been cutting community services, which means a lack of services in older people's own homes, which in turn means they are more likely to end up back in hospital.

This is absolutely absurd. 'There had been a huge emphasis on getting people out of hospital, rather than getting them out when they are ready,' said Help the Aged's public affairs head Kate Jopling.[13] 'There are huge problems about how older people are assessed and how much support is given, such as fitting homes with handrails or ensuring that people are on the right sort of medicines when they are sent home. If the system treated elderly people as individuals, this wouldn't be happening.'

Tackling this problem does require some cross-departmental thinking. Derby City Council arranges a community alarm installation and a support package for all older people on the day of their discharge. This is absolutely excellent, and hugely appreciated by the older people concerned and their families. It should not be beyond the wit of all local authorities to do something similar, and to make sure there is someone there at the end of the phone or alarm system if it goes off. I know how much this kind of system helped my parents and parents-in-law in the London Borough of Camden, where the service was impeccable over a period of eleven years.

But the evidence from Derby, which extended the provision of alarms to people living in all kinds of accommodation, private, council or housing association, was that they had created an effective multi-agency partnership between housing, social services, a registered social landlord and local NHS services.[14] That then led to an intensive rehabilitation service operating – for everyone – in a sheltered housing scheme. Doing this succeeded in massively reducing the numbers of falls and the incidence of hypothermia amongst older people over the age of 75, and reduced the numbers being admitted inappropriately to hospital or nursing home care.

When you read about it, it is blindingly obvious. It is also very uncommon, hence the Commission for Social Care Inspection's praise for the scheme. It is the complete opposite of the terrible case of a woman in Kent who was in a bed in an NHS hospital for more than four years after the doctors had said she was free to leave. This is thought to be the longest time a patient who has recovered has occupied a hospital bed, but it happened because there were no alternative care facilities available.[15] It probably cost the NHS more than £150,000 in total. That was a real disgrace, and it would have been so much easier for the NHS itself to set up the care facility it needed for patients like this.

The EverCare model, piloted by United Health in the USA, is another good example of what is possible.[16] This has an intensive programme of advanced primary nurses who do a great deal with older people at home, altering medication as necessary, bringing psychological support, responding rapidly in crises, and doing many of the things older people had been saying for years would make a difference – and which make them feel more secure. 'It gives me confidence because I can ring her anytime you know, any day, not like the doctors, and she'll come to me,' wrote one patient. Another one wrote: 'I don't bother with the doctors at all now; she sees to it all for me, for which I am most grateful. And doctors haven't too much patience with elderly people now.'

The only problem was that, unlike in the United States, the EverCare model as introduced into pilot sites in the UK does not reduce hospital admissions or indeed even lengths of stay insofar as the data can tell. So, though it was enormously popular with patients, carers and the nurses themselves, it did not make the difference that was expected. I suspect that it picked up a lot of unmet need out there, and also that our systems did not allow them to carry out the kind of intense interventions that would have stopped patients needing to go into hospital.

Policy responses

What might help more generally is simply better health care in old age, much as Muriel Gillick has been arguing so passionately in her books. A *British Medical Journal* editorial in 2006 said that national standards for the health, treatment and social care of older people in England – established in the national service framework (NSF) for older people back in 2001 – can be the basis of a way forward.[17] In April 2006, the UK's national director (the 'tsar') for older people, Professor Ian Philp, announced a set of new aims and targets in his report *A New Ambition for Old Age*.[18]

This set out eight standards to improve the experiences of older people and their carers who are using health, social care and other services. A standard on medicines management followed later, and then another ten programmes for implementing the framework, under three important and timely themes: dignity in care, joined-up care and healthy ageing.

The authors of the *BMJ* editorial, all senior doctors in the British Geriatric Society, argued that some things have improved since 2001, including more care being provided intensively in people's own homes, rather than in residential care.[19] They cited the reduction in delayed discharge from acute hospitals – the polite word for 'bed blocking'. They also suggested that specialist services for people with stroke and for those prone to falls are still improving. But they wanted new campaigns to promote greater physical fitness, reduce obesity, and provide for better management of sensory impairment and incontinence. Who organizes and runs these campaigns is irrelevant; they suggested voluntary organizations such as Age Concern and Help the Aged, supported by teams in primary and secondary care.

But the *BMJ* did argue that far too many of the targets set in the overall NHS plan are directed at younger people, and that the milestones and targets in the NSF for older people are largely ignored. It is true that Age Concern produces an excellent fact sheet for staying healthy in later life, but why isn't it available in every GP's surgery, or even widely disseminated in newspapers or even in the specialist older people's press, such as *Saga* magazine?

But the crux of their article was about money:

> *Other national service frameworks were supported with new monies, and despite older people being the prime users of primary care, secondary care, and social services*

*and having benefited from a reduction of four hour waits
on trolleys, investments have not been made in more
specific services such as general hospital care for older
people or an effective continence service ... Care for older
people is still not sufficiently integrated: it is sometimes
patchy, with limited progress against the framework's
targets, and with too many mismatches between needs
for and provision of care.*[20]

Their key accusation is that the increasing emphasis in the NHS on
moving patients rapidly through the emergency system towards
discharge – a hit-and-run approach – may well benefit younger people but, if it does so, it is at the expense of effective planning and
comprehensive specialist assessment of frail and old people. If you
mix in problems with community services, poor communication,
and disjointed planning between hospitals and the community, plus
the difficulty recruiting the right staff to work with older people,
then you have a serious problem.

Ian Philp's second report proposed new targets and protocols for
emergency responses to crises caused by falls, delirium, stroke and
transient ischaemic attacks.[21] One example is that everyone having
a stroke should be seen at a specialist neurovascular clinic within one
week, whilst the current position is that about half are seen by two
weeks. But the *BMJ* authors went much further, calling for 'appropriate environments' for care of older people, without 'multiple moves
between wards, and with timely discharge back to the community'.[22]

'Although intermediate care in the NHS is expanding,' they said,
'it is not yet keeping pace with the rapid and continuing closure of
rehabilitation beds and offers only patchy input from specialists.'

But despite all that rhetoric, the falls service has barely expanded
at all, even though a third of people over 65 fall each year, a fifth of

those over 80 fall each year, and many of them fall and cannot get up again. If they are not wearing an alarm of some kind, the problem is serious. Prevention is key, including exercising, especially T'ai Chi, which I talked about in Chapter 4.

The authors also argued that better co-ordination of care for people with complex needs can only be achieved by strengthening commissioning arrangements between the NHS and local authorities, to make sure that social care is not provided without medical problems being treated, by developing managed networks and building on successful developments in intermediate care. What we need is teams of health and social care providers to see, treat, help and review older people with complex problems, as set out in the primary care white paper.

They ended by saying that overt age discrimination is now uncommon in UK health and social care, but I'm not sure they are right. Professor Philp's *A New Ambition for Old Age* describes how some staff still show deep-rooted negative attitudes and negative behaviour towards older people, and it is overwhelmingly clear that older people feel that this discrimination exists.

Even the 'tsar' could see there was a problem: 'The dignity of older frail patients is infringed every day in many different ways. For example, in hospitals they are often asked to use bedpans and commodes behind curtains which provide inadequate privacy; not closing properly and allowing other people to see, hear, and smell what they are doing. The British Geriatrics Society has repeatedly expressed its concerns over this type of neglect, loss of dignity, and infringement of human rights.'[23]

Mental health

John Roberts, 84, spoke seven languages and was learning an eighth. Then Alzheimer's struck, as his daughter Yvonne described in the *Observer* in 2006:

> *He looks much as he did 20 years ago, except his beard had to go because it proved a trap for food when he was being fed. Last week the barber he had visited for years, but whom he no longer recognizes, shaved his cheeks bare – another small but necessary indignity that visibly marks the loss of his identity. One pitiful consolation is that he won't remember. My dad spent a lifetime in love with language – esoteric meanings, puns, poetry, jokes (often very blue), plus his own set of catchphrases that, just occasionally, could grate. How we long to hear them now. 'I've had an elegant sufficiency,' he would say with a flourish at the end of every celebratory meal. Now, he says little. He smiles occasionally as if to signal that his sense of humour, always strong, will be the last part of him to die.[24]*

But Yvonne Roberts explained something of what all that means to her mother, aged 82. 'Their plight is somewhat ignored, since they make few demands,' she wrote. 'They are the generation grateful to have survived the war and reared not to make a fuss, unlike their children ... So we have yet to comprehend fully the unrelenting scale of what is endured by sufferers and those who care for them. As a result, we also appear not to take too much notice. At least until, suddenly, it's not "old people" with Alzheimer's but our own mother and father. Or us.'

The cost of the drugs which can slow the process of the disease would be less than a place in a nursing home. The real question before NICE, says Yvonne Roberts, is 'precisely the one that society would prefer to avoid – are the elderly worth the money they require for a life worth living?'

The Alzheimer's Society estimates that dementia costs Britain £17 billion a year, and says that the government has no plan to deal with it. There are some 700,000 people suffering from dementia now, but the figure is expected to rise to more than a million in less than 20 years. Families bear the biggest burden, with carers saving the state some £6 biliion a year. But the cost of providing the same level of care to people suffering from dementia over the next 30 years is set to treble. Quite apart from anything else, many of those dutiful daughters who looked after their parents in previous generations now have high-flying careers or are locked into expensive mortgage repayments.

Dementia is also one of the main causes of disability in later life, well ahead of some forms of cancer, heart disease and stroke, yet much less is spent on research and care for sufferers. In fact, delaying the onset of dementia by five years would halve the number of deaths from dementia, saving 30,000 lives a year, but that seems to make no difference to the allocation of resources.

There is no doubt that better support to carers, and better skills across health and social care, would also make a huge difference, quite apart from picking up the tab for the cost of care for people who have severe dementia and can't be at home. The National Audit Office (NAO) published another searing report on dementia in 2007, and revealed that the Department of Health's programme board charged with improving things 'has not met for some time'.[25] The NAO was scathing about the fact that only a third to a half of dementia sufferers ever get a formal diagnosis, despite the fact that early diagnosis and intervention have been shown to be effective.

But the main debate has been about the use of drugs that are supposed to slow the progression of Alzheimer's disease. The UK's performance, according to the NAO, is in the bottom third in Europe, below almost all Northern and Western European nations.

Drugs are a real issue in the public mind. In November 2006, NICE (the National Institute for Clinical Excellence) issued guidance on dementia.[26] This was a drawn up together with the Social Care Institute for Excellence (SCIE) and was developed by the National Collaborating Centre for Mental Health, so it was hardly a swift, perverse piece of decision-making. The review panel included a patient representative, and there is no sense that NICE was not taking the arguments about Aricept and other drugs seriously. They just thought that there were other things that could be done that were more valuable. They may be right, but the proof of the pudding lies in whether services for people with Alzheimer's, which are often appalling, really improve as a result.

The guidelines pull no punches: 'As the condition progresses, people with dementia can present carers and social care staff with complex problems including aggressive behaviour, restlessness and wandering, eating problems, incontinence, delusions and hallucinations, and mobility difficulties that can lead to falls and fractures.'

It goes on to say that carers, care workers and healthcare professionals will have to be guided by the provisions of the Mental Capacity Act 2005, which came into force in 2007 and assumes that adults can make decisions for themselves, unless proved otherwise. It says that anything done for or on behalf of individuals without capacity must be the least restrictive alternative in terms of their rights and basic freedoms. This means that some of the restrictive practices – tying patients to their chairs, or using bucket chairs which older people can't get out of – are simply unacceptable under the new legislation.

The guidance goes on to emphasize how important it is that anyone with suspected dementia is seen by memory assessment services, including structural imaging to exclude other possible pathologies such as brain tumours or a subarachnoid haemorrhage. NICE suggests getting an MRI done, though they allow for the possibility of a CT scan as well. Yet thousands of people with dementia have never had anything like this, which suggests that doctors assume too quickly that the problem is dementia and that there is no other underlying cause for the symptoms.

The NAO report suggests that the development of memory services has been piecemeal and that services vary, even though 69 per cent of GPs have access to some kind of memory service. But although those services may exist, for some reason less than a third of GPs agree 'that there were satisfactory specialist services locally to meet the need'.[27]

The guidelines are extremely sensible, but some of their objectives are really no more than an ideal. The truth is that there are simply insufficient staff who are sufficiently highly trained to do much of this. Added to which, as any person with mild to moderate Alzheimer's disease will tell you, activities in which they are encouraged to take part are few and far between. All too frequently, activities specifically designed for older people ask people with Alzheimer's to stay away because they upset or confuse the other people there. Some voluntary sector organizations have set up specific daytime activities for people with Alzheimer's, but often those with more moderate symptoms rather resent being lumped together with those who have more severe disease, and resent being excluded from the activities designed for everyone else, young or old.

The NICE guidance goes into considerable detail about using drugs to treat, sedate or calm people with dementia who are aggressive or difficult, as well as suggesting that checks for depression and other physical causes of the behaviour, such as pain, are routinely made, which certainly doesn't happen now.[28] Despite the clear warnings about the use of such drugs, including a categorical statement on page 36 that healthcare professionals should monitor carefully for the 'emergence of severe untoward reactions, particularly neuroleptic sensitivity reactions ... particularly for patients with DLB (dementia with Lewy bodies)', there have since been a number of worrying cases of deaths as a result of just such prescriptions.

Nor is this new. Age Concern England produced guidelines for using neuroleptic drugs for older people with dementia back in 1998, which urged caution even before the more recent evidence was available, and suggested starting on very small doses and checking carefully for side-effects.[29] But the warnings were not taken seriously, as later stories in the press and elsewhere make clear.

In fact, research shows that people with Alzheimer's disease and other forms of dementia are twice as likely to die if they are prescribed neuroleptics, which are only being licensed for treating people with schizophrenia.[30] The research suggests they don't really help patients with milder symptoms, that they greatly increase their risk of dying prematurely, and yet 45 per cent of Alzheimer's patients in care homes are prescribed them. On average, patients who were on the drugs died six months earlier.

'If this was a massive increase in mortality in children there would be an outcry,' said the lead researcher, Clive Ballard, professor of age-related disorders at King's.[31] 'Older people aren't seen as a priority. These sedatives are being used because the services can't cope with people who are in a distressed state. There are ways to avoid them but it would involve training of staff, which is costly.'

Other aspects of the NICE guidelines are also detached from reality on the ground. They recommend that everyone with mild to moderate dementia should be given the opportunity to 'participate in a structured group cognitive stimulation programme ... commissioned by a range of health and social care staff with appropriate training and supervision, and offered irrespective of any drug prescribed for the treatment of the cognitive symptoms of dementia'. That really is wishful thinking. Activities like that are patchily available at best, and many of the patients find them impossible to attend or simply too frustrating.

Only after that did NICE set out their controversial guidance which suggests that only people with moderately severe Alzheimer's should be prescribed Aricept and the other acetylcholinesterase inhibitors. It was this decision, on top of what otherwise is very sensible and thorough guidance, though nowhere near the reality in practice, that has caused such an outcry with those with mild Alzheimer's and their carers.

In August 2007, the High Court ruled against an appeal that the manufacturers of the drug Aricept and the Alzheimer's Disease Society and other campaigners had brought against NICE's decision that Aricept's benefits in the early stages of Alzheimer's are too slight to justify prescribing it on the NHS. Actually, NICE got its decisions right in a difficult situation, since there is bound to be rationing in any health system. The questions that need to be asked are different ones about whether the facilities they assume are available for alternative treatments are actually in place.

But it is more complicated than that. If the benefit of Aricept for people in the earliest stages of Alzheimer's is slight, would the decision be different if the sufferers and those caring for them were younger? We can't know that, of course, but we can ask why rationing for those with Alzheimer's in the NHS is so tight that even the participative classes that NICE recommends barely exist.

Other mental problems

Only three days after the High Court ruling in August 2007, there was the publication of the report of the UK Inquiry into Mental Health and Well-Being in Later Life, chaired by Dr June Crown, herself a distinguished retired public health physician and former chair of Age Concern.[32] Once again, there was the dismal picture of a country with a mental health policy that focuses on those of working age, leaving older people with cheaper and often inferior care. It found that older people were given little or no help to cope with mental illnesses, and that vital care such as counselling is often withdrawn at the age of 65.

It is a familiar picture: health problems that were once taken seriously are simply dismissed as part of ageing, 'patronising and thoughtless' doctors dismissing debilitating conditions, with depression rarely treated in older people. According to the report, more than 3.5 million older men and women are denied adequate mental health care, and services are 'inadequate in range, in quantity and in quality'.

'Mental health problems in later life are not an inevitable part of ageing,' said Dr Crown. 'They are often preventable and treatable – and action to improve the lives of older people who have mental health problems is long overdue ... Our report draws attention to groups of older people who are currently invisible, who have been denied the fair treatment that should be the hallmark of a civilized society.'

The inquiry took place over a four-year period, and forecasts that the number of older people with mental health problems will grow by up to a third in the next 15 years. The cost to the economy will be enormous, with lost working days – if older people themselves, or their carers, are working – and lost buying power adding up to almost £500 billion annually by 2021. The mental health charity Mind said the report highlights the 'shameful neglect of older people who experience mental distress'.

The health minister Ivan Lewis responded by reminding people that the government had just announced a new national dementia strategy and was in the process of developing new guidelines for carers.[33] That strategy is all very well, but it is long overdue, as this plethora of shameful reports makes all too clear. 'We need to minimize the shame and fear associated with dementia so that people and their relatives feel able to seek support at the earliest possible stage in the knowledge they will get expert help and be treated with dignity and respect,' he said. Yet the lack of respect is something the government has knowingly presided over for a decade, and other governments, of other political persuasions, have done the same before it.

This is not about one government, or one political party. Their failure reflects just how little dementia is in the public's consciousness, and how low older people sit on the political priority list, and there is really no one to blame here but ourselves. If anyone is going to make it happen, we have to – backed by a ferocious grey power campaign that refuses to let ministers, officials and doctors off the hook.

Policy solutions

One of the peculiar aspects of all this is the way people are abused, even in the early stages of Alzheimer's disease, particularly if they are living alone. In the USA, it doesn't seem to matter that people have failed a test by doctors to put numbers in the right order on a clock, they can still be contacted by financial salesmen and sold wholly inappropriate products – 30 year mortgage deals at a fixed rate that end in their losing their homes – and the same could easily happen here if we are not careful.

The problem with the debate about whether specific drugs should be available is that it sidelines all this – as if one particular drug would magically transform the situation. Time and again, the NHS and social services have been criticized for the poor care offered to people with Alzheimer's and their carers. If this standard of care was offered to younger people with an ongoing, life-threatening, rapidly disabling disease there would be an outcry. Report after report has shown that the care is simply inadequate. Even worse than that, the kind of research that might be truly helpful – looking at social care interventions which might improve the quality of life for people caught in this situation – is in very short supply.

There isn't even much co-operation between health and social care services, which is so necessary for managing the mental health of older people. The National Audit Office found that only 29 per cent of Community Mental Health Teams had any joint health and social care funding arrangements.[34] The NAO report was fierce about what was needed, putting it very politely to the professions that they also need to get their houses in order and take these issues seriously. They are quite right. Many of the best, and most searing, reports on the state of older people's care come from the professions, or from others with heavy professional involvement. Yet the professionals themselves could, and should, do more to improve services rather than complain. This is not only a public policy matter, but one of professional leadership.

The NAO report also argues that local areas should commission a memory service where none exists, for those services to provide diagnosis along with advice and support, and referral to counselling as appropriate, and for acute hospital trusts to deal with the acute medical condition and then provide a mental health assessment as well, instead of saying it is nothing to do with them. But the most serious criticism, in a fiercely critical report, was reserved for the Department of Health, which it said should champion and co-ordinate improvements in dementia services as an explicit part of its approach to improving health and social care – and also think about running campaigns to raise awareness of dementia amongst front-line health and social care staff and the general public.

Although the UK compared reasonably with many of the other countries on some counts, it was doing far worse in comparisons over the prescription of drugs and its lack of a high-level policy initiative on dementia or older people's services more generally. This changed in August 2007, when the Department of Health finally launched theirs, but there is still a serious lag behind other countries, such as Australia, with its Department of Health and Ageing, and its ring-fenced programme of investment in dementia specific services, training and research. Other countries also provide more financial support for carers through, say, tax credits or social security allowances, and more employment-friendly policies to allow workers to take a period of paid leave to care for an older relative who is ill.

Home care for people with dementia

The UK Inquiry into Mental Health and Well-Being in Later Life made it clear that relationships were the most important thing: 'The main thing is love,' said Mrs W, 82, in their report.[35] 'Food, shelter, warmth are important, but it's the lack of someone caring that leads to despair.' Caring relationships are crucial to promoting and maintaining mental health and well-being, otherwise anything like the loss of a partner – which brings loneliness, isolation and loss – can all kick start poor mental health in older age.

'I object to being treated as a batty old age pensioner,' said one older woman, quoted by Mind's Access All Ages campaign.[36] 'Once you are a mental patient, that is all you are allowed to be. They strip you bare of any vestiges of culture, class, beliefs, education, experience of motherhood and grandmotherhood and what you might have achieved.'

Then there was Mick Fowell, 69, whose GP was quick to diagnose dementia 15 years earlier, but the follow-up mental health care was poor. He found most of the psychiatrists were 'trying to help but not really getting there'. He then used a drop-in bus service designed to reach rural locations like his home village of Gimingham, Norfolk. It proved a 'lifeline', in his terms, until it was axed in 2006. 'I shook the depression off after thinking, "If they don't help me, I am going to have to help myself",' he told the *Daily Mail*.[37] 'The bus going was the final straw, but I have always been angry because I have seen the deterioration of mental health services on an almost daily basis.'

It is in these early stages of mental problems in old age that local authorities seriously fail the carers and the patients. The systems are not in place, even if they were once before. The staff are not available, which stores up problems for later, which might be considerably more expensive. The Crown report cites clear evidence that what older people with mental health problems really want is a 'person-centred' approach that allows them to be treated as individuals who can be involved in decisions about their care, rather than being told what they have to do.[38] They want support, respect, equal access, choice and involvement in decision-making. It really isn't much to ask.

Nor is all this about dementia. Many older people suffer from depression for all sorts of reasons. Yet it is all too often ignored, as Mary Godfrey makes only too clear in her work for Help the Aged.[39] The prevalence of depression amongst those in care homes is two to three times higher than it is in the wider community, at about 40 per cent. It is more common in women than in men, and is caused by a variety of factors, including disability and bereavement, but it is also eminently treatable. The trouble is that, when it is combined with mild dementia, it is often not even noticed.

What makes this so infuriating is that many aspects of the care of older people with mental health problems are getting worse in the UK. Local authorities are cutting back on eligibility to services as part of their cost-cutting measures, which is very serious for people with dementia and their often very elderly carers. They could also take more responsibility for making sure the quality of care workers coming into people's homes is high enough, even if they don't themselves provide the care. After all, those who receive the services are often too vulnerable to be able to deal with difficulties themselves. The NAO's web forum on the issue talked about home care being rushed 'as if on a conveyor belt'.

In fact, seven out of ten local authorities can now only afford to provide care to people with the most critical needs. If this increasing trend of rationing services carries on then, by as early as 2009, no older people will get care until their needs reach this substantial/critical level, and even then it will probably continue to be poor quality and rushed.

In theory, anyone who is over 16 and provides essential care for a friend or relative is entitled to a Carer's Assessment. That is supposed to let them discuss what support they need to care for someone, and to maintain their own health, and to balance caring with their life, work and family commitments. That is all very fine and dandy, but social services have been setting eligibility criteria on the basis of available funding. That means that, even if carers have identified needs, nothing may be provided for them if their needs are not judged severe enough, according to the local authority's own criteria. The result is that tens of thousands of families, often wives and husbands, are being left to care for frightened, often difficult, older people with dementia, and – because of a shortage of cash, and an emphasis on protecting younger people – the money simply isn't there to stop the total breakdown of family care by early intervention.

The tragedy is that, without those carers, the financial burden on those same local authorities would be considerably greater. Yet all the evidence is there that shows early intervention is extremely helpful, and is valued by people with dementia themselves and their families,

One study found that care staff themselves felt the most useful part of their training had been the modules which improved their understanding of depression in the residents, which had made them more tolerant, less judgemental and more able to make sense of behaviour and problems. Good training can, in other words, lead to better communication and more autonomy and independence for older people.

Depression

There is an urgency about this. There is widespread public policy attention given to the high suicide rates among young men, and the national suicide prevention strategy aims to cut suicide rates by high-risk groups by 20 per cent by 2010. Yet by far the highest risk group is older people. The highest rate of all suicide attempts is amongst the over-65s, and one in four attempts results in a death, compared with one in 30 in the general population. Yet the evidence suggests that neither policy-makers, nor those who provide care to older people, realize there is a problem – either that or they are simply not acting on it. Quite the reverse. Professionals often describe depression as somehow 'normal' in old age, as if it was ever 'normal' to feel depressed.

Older people are given little access to mainstream mental health services, including psychological therapies – such as cognitive behaviour therapy with its proven track record in treating depression – and support groups. At best, they get given anti-depressants. At worst, they are over-treated with pill after pill, with little other support, and at the very worst they get nothing at all. No surprise, then, that they become suicidal. One study suggests that between a half and two thirds of those suicides could be avoided if depression in people over 65 was adequately treated.[40] But, in order to achieve that, there would need to be a complete rethink of mental health services for older people, from dementia to depression, and everything in between.

What might that mean? Apart from better services across care homes, nursing homes and in older people's own homes, and a wider duty on society to take care of isolated older people, there may be a role for community nurses who specialize in old age, such as the specialist nurses for older people at home put forward as a possibility by Hazel Heath for the Clore Duffield Foundation.[41] Their role would be to spot isolation and mental distress.

It also means thinking outside the box, using music and the arts to help support people who are suffering from dementia. It means coming up with social innovations that can provide the support and relationships people need, not just more reliance on technology or pharmaceuticals.

West Berkshire Alzheimer's Society runs a 'Singing for the Brain' programme which uses music to stimulate communication, given that musical abilities are often the last to be lost in cases of severe brain damage or degeneration. This works to stimulate communication for people who have largely lost the capacity, as well as getting them out of the house. Singing also helps them enjoy better physical health; music stimulates the hormones that help to regulate sleep patterns and aggressive behaviour in older people. The Sidney de Haan Research Centre for Arts and Health is developing a participatory singing activity programme for older people, including those suffering from dementia.

It works, but it is still so rare.

Poor hospital care

Probably the most shocking evidence of what is happening to older people is the bulging cuttings files devoted to their care in hospital, often brought to light by campaigns being led, amongst others, by the *Daily Mail*, the *Observer* and Help the Aged. Some have focused on nutrition, some on the low level of care by care assistants. Most are about how old people's needs, particularly those with dementia towards the end of their lives, are simply ignored.

Take the story of Ros Levenson's mother, set out in the *British Medical Journal* in 2006, who was in hospital with trouble swallowing.[42] She was asleep most of the time, and the speech and language therapists said she was to be 'nil by mouth'. The staff could not get a nasogastric tube into her, and said she would need a PEG (percutaneous gastrostomy tube) so she could be fed. Ros Levenson knew her mother would not want that, but the staff persisted because – or so it appeared – this was standard practice, so she discussed it with the consultant, who seemed to agree.

Ros' mother then seemed more awake, so she asked if they could try her on swallowing again. 'I was told there were 28 patients and two nurses and they did not have the time,' she said. 'I had to say that I had only one mother and she had no one to look out for her but me, and I insisted on the assessment being made.'

The assessment was made with no result, then – about 20 days after admission to hospital – one of the nurses asked her if she would reconsider and allow a PEG to be put in, because 'it might give her a chance'. Ros disagreed. She clarified it with the doctors, who said they had not wanted a PEG. The nurses refused to try to feed her manually because they said she couldn't swallow, and on it went. This went on: the speech therapists said no, the nurses said no, the doctors said try manual feeding, and it seemed as if they were back to square one.

'The nurses found it very difficult to care for a patient without doing what they considered was everything possible to lengthen life,' Ros wrote. 'They also found it hard to be in a situation where they feared personal blame.'

In 2005, the nurse Margaret Haywood worked undercover for the BBC programme *Panorama* for three months, recording her experience of an acute medical ward. 'The memory that will haunt me for the rest of my life is of a lady who was terminally ill with cancer crying out in pain because she hadn't been given her pain relief on time,' she wrote later.[43] 'That was just so heartbreaking it really did upset me. When I did a couple of shifts in a row, I was able to make sure she did get her pain relief on time and the change in her was sometimes quite remarkable. There was no good reason why it hadn't been given to her.'

People who needed help to eat were often not getting it, some patients were thirsty and some were without proper night clothes, in gowns open at the back. Patients were not getting their medication and, if it had been like that when she started nursing, she said she would have left.

When Peter Coles, chief executive of that same hospital, was shown the footage before broadcast and was interviewed by the BBC, he was disturbed and shocked, and apologized on behalf of the trust for what he had seen.[44] He said they had received complaints the previous year and had put in place 'a whole series of changes on the ward culminating in a new ward manager'. But he could find no answer to the specific problems – a woman waiting for two hours to be taken to the toilet when nursing guidelines say five minutes, a woman crying out with pain with terminal cancer, and so on, just that what was seen was unacceptable. And it was. When asked what priority the care of elderly people had in his hospital, Coles assured the interviewer: 'It has a high priority.'

The bottom line was that this was a ward for older people and standards were shockingly low, so that people died without being noticed, without a friend being asked to come and be with them and hold their hands. There was pain, soiling, failure to toilet people, and patients left in bed all day. Worse, it wasn't that unusual.

Four of the patients featured in the *Panorama* programme died before it was broadcast, and one of the nicest things was seeing a short obituary of each of them on the programme's website – Ivy Constable who died aged 96, in hospital; Jessie Mowitt, who used to work for the International Labour Organization in Geneva and chose Brighton so she could get to London's galleries easily; Gwenda Thackray, who died of liver cancer in hospital. Also Hilda Burnham, who had herself been a nurse, who thought long and hard about what care should be like, and who approved of the undercover *Panorama* reporting.

She told one of the reporters what she thought made a good nurse: 'Being able to feel in your own heart what the patient is feeling. You can't nurse and be indifferent to your patients. No matter how you try not to, they become interwoven into your life.' She returned home after being filmed in hospital but died shortly afterwards, on a hospital trolley in A&E, in January 2005.

Other stories make the blood boil. Like Martin Bright's grandmother, Irene Emmings, in a Bath hospital who, unable to speak, left notes by her bed detailing the neglect and abuse she had endured.[45] Or there was Jane Kerr's aunt, Ruby, whose food was whisked past her if she was asleep. 'Today her fingernails are thick with dirt or excrement, her blonde hair is unwashed and unbrushed and, when I arrive mid-morning, she is lying on a pad soaked in urine ... and balance this with the knowledge that Ruby was only admitted with dehydration and a urinary tract infection after staff at her home noticed she had a raised temperature,' wrote Jane in the *Daily Mirror*.[46]

Three days later she fell and damaged her hip, and then wasn't moved for five weeks. The problem was that the nurses couldn't move her until they knew whether her hip had been fractured, and they wouldn't know that until the X-ray results came through.

Surely the X-ray results would come back right away. No, the nurse explained that the X-rays can't just go to Ruby's doctor, they have to be referred to a specialist orthopaedic surgeon for his verdict. This took three weeks, and then it turned out her hip wasn't fractured after all, so Jane Kerr tried to get her up because her care home would have her back if she could stand. Her carer, Arthur, persisted in trying to get her out of bed, but one of the nurses said: 'I wouldn't do that if I were you ... she has loose bowels and I'll have to mop up.'

In fact, the 28 patients in the ward were all suffering from severe diarrhoea and sickness, and were being told to drink as much as they could. But they couldn't, because the cups were placed out of reach. When Jane complained, two nurses tried to wash Ruby between the legs – she had been lying in her own excrement; the cries were pitiful as she felt she was being attacked, but no one had time to reassure her. And this was the former headmistress, an intelligent, gentle, immaculately turned-out woman.

In October 2007, a few days after the shocking revelations about 90 older people having died in the care of Maidstone and Tunbridge Wells NHS trust as a result of *clostridium difficile*, where the care was shocking and old people were left lying in their own excrement, the *Observer* published an investigation into a more general feature on the wards, about how elderly people are often left by overworked staff to soil their beds.[47] What it showed was that care staff no longer routinely accompany older patients to the toilets, instead advising them to go in the beds. So shocking did this seem, with rising complaints about older people being stripped of their dignity, that Ivan Lewis, the minister responsible, warned that staff would face negligence charges if found guilty of providing seriously substandard care.

The problem is that this warning is not enough. How did we get into this position? The British Geriatric Society has rightly launched a campaign, Behind Closed Doors, to highlight the bad practice it wants to see banned. Their warnings 'suggest that for many patients the prospect of having to relieve themselves using a commode on a mixed sex ward with only a thin curtain round the bed is one of the main reasons why they fear going into hospital'. The *Observer* article continued with Jackie Morris, chair of the society's policy group, listing practices which she argues 'most people would find it hard to believe hospital chief executives still allow':

> *Patients who need the toilet are being told to wait maybe for an hour or more. Patients can often hear a person who is forced to use a commode. It's a fundamental part of dignity, that you should be able to relieve yourself in private. But you often see this vicious cycle happening where patients who may be recovering from an operation are not taken to the loo, but instead given a commode or even told to go in their pants.*[48]

Quite apart from the pressure sores this can cause, which are painful and scary, this can also lead to patients refusing to eat and drink because they become scared of needing to go to the loo. All of which suggests a disgraceful lack of consideration of what it must feel like – a lack of empathy from staff who will themselves be old one day, if they do not die first.

Food

Food and drink are a constant source of complaint. Bert Webster, 77, was admitted to hospital with a lung infection, following a fall at home, weighing just seven stone (44.3 kg).[49] During a three-month stay in a hospital in North London he lost another 2 kg from his spare frame, despite his vulnerable condition – he had also recently had a stroke and was battling vascular dementia. His daughter, Lisa MacMurdie, said his meals would just be left on his tray, even though he was unable to cut up his food, let alone eat it. He said the only support he got to eat was from visiting relatives, and that meant he would often go hungry. Bert's weight should have been monitored weekly, but this didn't happen either.

Being confused, Bert would try to feed himself with a knife, or spoon food into the bed. On one occasion he soiled himself as he had become so miserable and confused, and all that happened then is that the clothes he was wearing at the time were taken off him and dumped under his bed, and remained there for several days, until Lisa discovered them by chance when she came to visit him.

In the results of a survey conducted over 2005/6, families were finding that they had to turn up at the hospitals to feed their older relatives and make sure they didn't go without.[50] Dieticians give advice on what to eat for certain conditions, but here they are needed more generally. The emphasis on food needs to grow, and more needs to be spent on the food itself, and on those who prepare it, serve it and help frail people eat it. We need tempting dishes, attractive to those who are to eat them, according to their tastes. That is probably more important than the appalling pushing of a plug into the stomach, where food – a different form of gloop – can be poured straight in, without the need to help a frail and vulnerable person to eat in the normal way.

It may seem easier for staff to feed a patient that way, particularly an older person who has all sorts of reflexes that make them liable to choking and coughing. But eating is one of life's great pleasures. You get nothing from gloop poured into the stomach except a sense of being replete – no pleasure, no sense of satiety, no anticipation, no sense of community with others eating at your table. It is just a quick, hi-tech fix. It isn't eating. It is as if staff have lost sight of the importance of a basic human function, not only because feeding older patients takes time, but because many of them may have relatively little experience of sitting at a table in a civilized way with family all around, eating together, as that becomes less and less common in society at large.

But then, as the old people's tsar Ian Philp said: 'Things happen to older people that, if they happened to children, would end up in the criminal courts.'[51]

Call to arms

There are any number of cases like these, amounting to punishment and neglect for being old, and they are immensely distressing. But the problem is not wholly new, and the *British Medical Journal* drew attention to the ageism in the NHS back in 1999.[52] Assistant editor Alison Tonks argued that older people faced arbitrary discrimination in their encounters with health professionals, which probably reflects a wider ageism within society. They were excluded from research and many beneficial interventions, some of which would be life-saving, and were insensitively managed. She said that recent changes in acute medical services in Britain had created an environment where ageism flourished: more and more older people are now admitted to fewer and fewer beds for shorter and shorter stays.

Nearly a third of beds for acute cases are now occupied by people over 75, and the throughput per bed over the past 10 years in the geriatric sector has more than doubled. Whilst the health needs of most older people are the same as they are for everyone else, the 'oldest old' and those with chronic diseases or disability, are characterized by multiple pathology, non-specific presentations, have a high incidence of secondary complications, and need intensive rehabilitation. They need a generalist approach to assessment and treatment and are poorly served by a super-specialist profession. Even doctors who specialize in caring for older people often prefer curing acute illnesses to using their skills in chronic disease and rehabilitation. To combat age discrimination health professionals and their institutions must acknowledge it, document it and then act to eradicate it, said the *BMJ*.

Tonks talked about partnerships with older people to enhance core teaching, and giving older health service users the power to actually shape the curriculum of professionals. Later on, all doctors could get the necessary skills by doing six months in geriatric medicine during training. 'Reshaping the health service around older patients need not be painful and can start now,' said Tonks:

> *Even small adjustments to the ward, clinic, or surgery can make a difference. For example, admission wards with access to a breadth of expertise are better for patients with multiple problems than direct admission to a specialist (say orthopaedic) ward. Individual doctors can also make a difference by seeking out and removing their own prejudices. More sweeping changes will have to follow, however, including: engaging older people in the commissioning and design of services; accepting that undergraduate and postgraduate training produces doctors whose aspirations don't match the needs of their patients; finding and protecting money to pay for care of older people; returning to an emphasis on rehabilitation and convalescence; and changing the way we think. If the health service could be made fit for older people, it would be fit for everybody.*

Unfortunately, right now, it really isn't fit for everybody, and older people are treated worst of all. We need nurses who can see that, care assistants who are paid enough and respected enough to change things, and an attitudinal shift that makes leaving old people lying in their own faeces, or in intolerable pain, simply unacceptable to any staff member at all.

We need to tackle this general lack of concern for older people at both ends. One end is this endemic sense, throughout our healthcare system, that older people are worth less. There remain pockets of the NHS where this isn't the case – what community nurses do is often absolutely brilliant – but the giveaway is the increasing reference inside the system to older people as 'bed blockers', as if it was their fault. The question is how much this refers to older people as a nuisance just because they are 'blocking' beds, or whether it carries within it an implication that they are more fundamentally nuisances. As if they were somehow unnecessary people. Either way, the more that attitude is voiced inside the NHS, the more staff are infected by it, and the more their own negative impression of older people is legitimized.

We can and must tackle those attitudes with better training and with legislation to outlaw ageism. But we can also tackle the problem at the other end. Older people may sometimes be occupying acute beds which they no longer need quite so badly, but if there are no convalescent beds for them to move to, and if the community hospitals have closed and they would otherwise be going home to an empty house, what are they supposed to do? The system has removed the institutions which would have been valuable to them and is now blaming them for it. So it makes sense to rebuild that infrastructure. **The NHS needs to recreate its network of convalescent beds and community hospitals, and support at home – bolstered by a new generation of mutual volunteer support – to help older people recover after hospital stays.**

What remains of the community health system still provides good care for older people. Many GPs, community nurses and primary care centres do a very good job for them. The problems come when they need any kind of moderately acute health intervention and go into hospital – as people do at any age – and then the system collapses, especially when the time comes for them to come out again. We need community beds, not just for older people, but for anybody with a long-term condition, to get people back to a position where they can manage reasonably on their own. Public policy mouths these truths about the importance of community care and home care, but in practice the basic connections are still not being made.

The manifesto also needs to include demands to:

- **End discrimination in healthcare.** There will always have to be some kind of rationing in the NHS, but it is indefensible that this should be done on the basis of age, so that older people are always at the end of the queue, always get the cheapest solutions – where they get them at all – and never see the specialists they need. A health system based on that kind of discrimination, for whatever reason, is inhuman – and it leads to far worse cruelties that are inflicted on older people on the wards. In particular, we need to guarantee speedy, expert treatment to older stroke victims.

- **Build relationships back into the healthcare system.** There is still fantastic care for older people available in primary care, and from many GPs who build relationships with their older patients, rather than simply applying technocratic policy to their cases, as hospital trusts tend to do. The drift to large polyclinics, where patients rarely see the same doctor twice, is unlikely to be as effective for older people, because those relationships with individual GPs are important. They are particularly helpful when older patients have a range of interlocking conditions, when seeing the same person will help prevent dangerous drug interactions and pick up on very small changes which may be quite significant.

- **Send trainee health professionals to live with a family of someone with a long-term condition.** Many professionals have no experience of this at all, then they go into training, pick up these widespread attitudes towards older people, but haven't got the personal experience they need to counter the influence. Young people in training need a dose of what it feels like from an older person's perspective, before they imbibe the attitudes that are in the paint in the NHS.

- **Build joint teams that link health and social care in every local authority.** We need some serious cross-departmental thinking, not just community alarms and support packages for all older people on the day of their discharge from hospital, but an end to the squabbling over resources that delays and undermines the home care of so many older people around the country.

Chapter 9

Don't treat my death as meaningless

The right to die well

Death, like grandchildren, is one of the extraordinary and exciting perks of old age. Over 60, it's time to get acquainted with it. No use dreading it, or being frightened by it. People are always wringing their hands when their friends die, but, frankly, what did they expect? That they'd live forever?

Virginia Ironside, *Independent,* **19 September 2006**

That urge to stay young will eventually, with good fortune, transmute into a benign acceptance that life can't go on for ever. That's the most we can hope for. The prospect of dying frightens some ... [but] I favour the more sentimental Walter Savage Landor: 'I fought with none for none was worth my strife/Nature I loved and next to nature art/I warmed my hands before the fire of life/It sinks and I am ready to depart.' Not just yet, though. The embers are still glowing.

Joan Bakewell, *Guardian,* **19 August 2005**

'My father was cared for on and off for the last few years of his life by staff in the cardiology ward of the Royal Free Hospital in Hampstead. He always joked that he had been in every ward of the Royal Free except the maternity wards, but in fact most of his admissions were to cardiology, and they knew him well there. After the difficult conversation I had with him, passing on what the doctor had said – that it might not be sensible to simply patch him up again – several nurses spent a great deal of time talking to him, asking him how he felt about dying, and asking him what his wishes were.

He trusted the staff there because of an incident some time before. He had decided to discharge himself from hospital on a bank holiday Sunday – why is the NHS so hopeless over bank holidays? – before they could set up any support at home, and a nurse and a young doctor spent hours in the freezing cold, as he sat in my car threatening to drive away, persuading him to stay until care could be organized. One nurse in particular, Ann Hamlet, befriended him and got his confidence completely, so that he could tell her things he felt he could not tell us.

When he did come home, for what turned out to be the last 28 hours of his life, everyone involved was enormously kind and helpful, from the ambulance men who carried him upstairs and teased him, to the wonderful district nurse who took charge of the situation and helped us organize the next few days, to the Marie Curie nurses who came to be with him constantly, to the GP who helped the district nurse make his bed, and was kindness itself to my mother and me. It was a team effort between professionals and across organizations of a quality I had not witnessed before at such close quarters. It was also an object lesson, as a carer, of how much difference really professional staff can make when they care passionately about what they do.

My father was a very large man, and it took two or three people to turn him. So we had a visit from the night community nurses, one of whom spent quite some time comforting me. Despite her working in the NHS trust I chaired, I had never met her before. I decided I would certainly go out with them one night, and watch that remarkable service from a more objective standpoint. I was fascinated by the considerable comfort they were able to bring, late at night when the world is silent, and early in the morning when fears run highest.

When it became clear that my father was sinking fast, and Alison the district nurse, and Carol the Marie Curie nurse, helped me make it clear to my mother – though she didn't really accept it at the time – the way they did it was a lesson in how to provide care and support, to my father, my mother and to me. Carol even took my son home at the end of her shift. It was well beyond the call of duty.

I wish it was always like this. People might say it was as a result of privilege, because I chaired the trust, that we were treated so well. But I am so old that I changed my name when I got married. My father and I didn't share a surname and, though some of the staff knew who I was, the engaging young man who came to collect the equipment from Home Loans certainly hadn't got a clue, and his smiling face and considerable charm as he expressed his sympathies were helpful in themselves.

When I told him that the wheelchair had originally been delivered to my office and was now going back with him, and asked him to explain it to Cath, he looked at me quizzically and asked how I knew Cath. I explained that I chaired the trust, at which he seemed completely unfazed, and just said – quite correctly – that I didn't look the same as I did in my photographs. That was not entirely surprising after the exhaustion of three days and nights in the same pair of jeans, and such a roller-coaster of emotions.

It was only a few weeks later that my father-in-law died at home, and was also looked after by some of our district nurses. There the name was the same as mine, but everyone by then knew that he was not my father. Once again, the care was remarkable. He had private nurses as well, and the integration between NHS and private worked extraordinarily well. The district nurses provided great comfort to my father in-law, but also remarkable support to my mother-in-law, husband, brother-in-law and the rest of the family. Once again, it was a faultless service. Once again, an older man died in his own home, surrounded by loved ones, pain-free and peacefully, just as he and his family had hoped.

I know it isn't always like this. I hear all too often about parts of the country, even parts of London, where such care is not made available, where the palliative care service doesn't cover weekends, or really provide a proper service integrated with the community nurses. But our experience was quite wonderful. It left us all with a feeling of deep gratitude, of wonder at the devotion of the people who provide that service day after day to very distressed people, and also quite certain that we should provide this for everybody, everywhere, throughout the country.'[1]

The journalist Melanie Phillips described a similar experience in the Jewish care home where her mother died. She was in a partial coma when the aromatherapist arrived and gently applied her oils and whispered words of encouragement:

> She sprinkled fragrant essences on her pillows and put on
> the soft soothing background music that my mother had
> come to love in the years in which she had drawn comfort
> from this treatment. Nor was this all. The aromatherapist
> took a quick lunch and then came back and did it all over
> again ... She understood, from her care of that body, that

what was ending here was a monumental struggle. And
what was so moving was that, even though my mother
could not respond, and, for all we knew, was quite
unaware of what was going on, she was treated right to
the end as a person with particular likes and desperate
needs; and, even more touchingly, as if she was still as
alert and responsive as she had always been. It was a
reaffirmation of humanity.[2]

When the NHS or the care homes get it right, it seems to me, we need to shout about it much more loudly, show it to other countries where people still die hospitalized deaths attached to tubes. But before we do that, we need to make sure it is possible for everyone here in the UK to receive that kind of care as well.

One key feature of all the interviews I carried out for this book, not to mention the unofficial conversations, walking up hills and down mountainsides with friends, was how we think about death. Most of the older people I know – and by that I mean people from their fifties onwards – seem remarkably unscared of dying.

My father was deeply upset when he learned there was nothing else that the doctors could do for him, but I don't think he was scared. He just wanted to go home. My mother was certainly not scared, but she would neither talk about it nor acknowledge that dying was what she was about. Friends and family talk openly about dying, where they want to be, and how they want to do it. There is no doubt that older people know death is coming, and their fear is very often not so much of death itself, but of being warehoused in a hospital that can do little for them or a nursing home where they will be expected to still sit and wait.

But there are some people who are still scared, and that fear is undoubtedly something we need to deal with. The writer and director Jonathan Miller reflected on this with great sensitivity:

> Yes, there are specific dyings that I'm frightened of but
> the fear of just not existing? No, I don't have that at all. I
> suppose every now and then, in a sort of sentimental,
> paranoid, Housmanesque way: 'Is my team ploughing?' –
> you know? The idea that the place will close over, and
> that other people whom I thought I was fond of and were
> fond of me will in fact get on with their lives. It's
> connected, I think, with something which was very early
> in childhood, at the age of about seven or eight – frosty,
> wonderful, welcoming Christmas parties, and of being
> collected slightly early, of there still being musical chairs,
> and of having to go before musical chairs, and jellies ...
> It's being taken into the darkened hall, and the lights are
> on in the room, and half glimpsed there's a pretty girl
> crossing a lighted doorway, in an organdie dress, and
> laughing en route to some festivity that one now can't
> have.[3]

There is no doubt, also, that some people's experience of death includes something which can only be described as beautiful. Diana Athill describes her mother's death like that:

> When the time came for my mother to die, she was
> almost unbelievably lucky – and therefore I was too. On
> the day before her 96th birthday she walked on her two
> sticks down to the end of her garden to oversee the
> planting of a new eucalyptus tree by Sid Pooley. Halfway

through the planting he thought she looked not quite herself. 'Are you all right?' he asked, and she said she was feeling a bit unsteady and had better go back to the house. He helped her back, settled her in her chair, and called Eileen Barry, her home help, who recognized heart failure when she saw it. Ellen got her to the local cottage hospital and called me – by then it was 8.30 in the evening – saying it would probably be a good thing if I got there first thing next morning: no, she didn't think it was necessary for me to come straight away ...

The actual moment of death was so extraordinary that she wrote a poem about it afterwards called 'The Gift'. It was difficult, behind screens in a crowded ward, with her mother vomiting into a basin, but she was conscious, and – when Diana put her hand in hers – there was a 'great flash' of recognition and joy. 'It was the love I had never doubted flaming into visibility,' wrote Diana. 'I *saw* what I had always believed in ...'[4]

Facing death clearly

My mother-in-law, of an earlier generation, also talked about 'leaving the party' before it was over, but her wish was to go before life became meaningless and painful which, by and large, she achieved – and after a wonderful life. She rejoiced in the sense that life would go on, that her children and grandchildren would live full and busy lives, but she didn't want to prolong the dying. The point is that people talk about it, and need to do so, despite the fact that it remains a taboo subject in many care homes. Marjorie Reeday, a resident of the Simon Marks Court care home near Leeds, is busy planning her own funeral.[5] 'I want to have the service in our lounge,' she told the

Guardian in 2006. 'There's been a death recently and it was a beautiful service. It wasn't depressing; it was joyful. I want mine to be like that.'

Staff at her care home advised Marjorie how to make a will and how to make her own funeral arrangements. She talked quite openly with her carers about her fears about her own death. 'I want to leave my body to medical research,' she said. 'I've talked it over with them here and they're helping me to fill in the forms.'

This is such a welcome change from the usual atmosphere in care homes. The gerontologist Malcolm Johnson argues that it is the care staff who find it embarrassing and difficult to talk about, not the residents.[6] 'By hiding the reality and giving them no opportunity to talk about it, we are doing them a real disservice,' he said.

So Anchor Homes came up with the plan, working with Johnson, to give staff training courses to approach death in a sensitive manner. It has changed a variety of things, including interestingly in one home where the residents made it clear they didn't like the bodies being taken out the back door. 'We came in though the front door so we want to go out by the front door,' they said. Nor did they like the body bags the undertakers used, so they made a cover in the crafts area to cover the bodies as they left. They also have a memory board pinned up now, with memories of the residents who had died recently pinned up to help the bereaved people mourn. This is a massive change from the reluctance to look death in the eye and face what is coming.

There is, in fact, some kind of change in the air about our attitude to death. More and more books on the subject have been published and academic 'thanatology' has become a subject students can study. Several authors have wanted to take on the death taboo, from Kate Berridge with her sparkling *Vigor Mortis*, dedicated to the dear departed, to Help the Aged's superb *End-of-life Care* volume, subtitled 'Promoting comfort, choice and well-being for older people', and written by Jane Seymour and others.[7]

But not only did they publish a guide to making it better, they also published a magnificent volume entitled *Dying in Older Age,* with reflections and experiences from an older person's perspective.[8] In it, older people talk about how they face their own mortality. Margaret Buzan, 88, talked about tidying her paperwork so that her two sons don't have too much to do. She has left a list of presents she has already bought to give to people, so they can pass them on. She has told them when she has booked tickets for the theatre or whatever in advance and where the tickets are, so they can know what the show is and, if she dies before the show date, they can take someone else.

It is all beautifully thought through, very practical, but based on a strong desire not to be leaving a mess behind. Margaret also said she discusses all this not only with friends but, more surprisingly, with acquaintances. She volunteers at a day centre for physically handicapped older people and has often managed to talk to them about death and dying. She mentioned a 93-year-old lady in great pain who had been told she needed surgery, but the anaesthetists had said her heart was weak and she might not survive. She had opted for the surgery, after a good long life. 'I think in her position I would feel likewise,' said Margaret.

Or there was George Fullwood, a retired engineer, who said it was important that we realize that 'everyone dies alone. It is addressing all the fears and making choices and putting your affairs in order that you need to do with other people before you go.'

Or Nan Maitland, founder of Homeshare, and a social worker and care manager by career, who really would prefer autonomy in her death. She supports Dignitas, the organization in Switzerland that allows physician-assisted suicide, and she clearly feels horrified by old, decaying bodies:

> *I am certainly not going to wait around for God. I have arthritis now and many relatives with dementia, so that means I have a good chance of getting dementia and my arthritis will certainly get worse. I also have a strong constitution, no heart problems, low blood pressure, low cholesterol, none of the killer diseases, and healthy long-lived parents; so the actuarial tables say I am likely to live till 103. I am determined that I am not going to end up demented and with every movement agony ... at that point I want to be in control and say: 'Enough is enough. Goodbye.' The law must be changed so that those who wish to can end their lives when they want to do so in comfort.*

And there was Margaret Simey, the wonderful political campaigner and councillor in Toxteth for 23 years. Her take on old age was less than happy – she died shortly after the interview – but what she said struck home:

> *I can't stand the crushing boredom of the life I now lead, busy though it keeps me. When all the days are the same, it is no wonder I can't remember what day of the week it is, let alone what month. I am weary of being grateful for the gift of a bunch of bananas or a custard tart when I am starving for something to think about. I live on the brink of not being able to manage ... and if I can't manage, is there anybody there to rescue me? The answer, I suspect, will be 'We don't do that.'*

She saw herself as two people, one who is incapacitated whom she dubs the Old Cow, the other the outgoing sociable person with masses of interests whom she regards as her real self.

This new openness about death has extended to some of the big charities. Quite apart from the thriving hospice movement itself, the Marie Curie charity is doing a great deal to change how primary care handles death at home, and the New Philanthropy Capital think-tank has published *Caring about Dying* to help philanthropists who want to support this area of better dying.[9] The *British Medical Journal* managed a whole issue on dying back in 2003, and there are now national minimum standards in what people can expect when they die.[10] There is also an increasing academic interest in death and dying, which helps get the subject out of the shadows, brought to life by people such as the wonderful Peter Jupp – who wrote *Death in England: An Illustrated History* with Clare Gittings, back in 1999 – who has helped run and edit the journal *Mortality* for well over a decade.[11] All this is shifting the subject from the unspeakable to an area of interest, even if it is still of limited interest. It is not enough, but it is a huge improvement.

So there is a sense of ending, and some fear, but more because of the pain, discomfort and sadness around death than the actual dying. Partly this may be because so many of us no longer believe – whatever our faith or none – in a real after-life, and certainly not in a final Day of Judgment when we will be held personally to account. That old 'religious' fear, a form of religious terror, is not real for most of us in the West. What does remain is the wish to convey our lives and record ourselves, and to make an impact, especially as – for so many of us – our immortality will lie in what is left behind us.

Sorting things out

In the Jewish tradition, there is an old custom, being somewhat reinvented now, of leaving ethical wills for our children. I had great fun asking some well-known people to write an ethical will for their descendants to be broadcast on Radio 4 some years ago, and it was very enlightening. What we want to leave behind is so often our values, the feeling that we have influenced people, enhanced lives, comforted sorrows and provided a strong moral code for our children.

This kind of will has its roots in the medieval period, but it applies just as much now. This is a seventeenth-century example of the ethical will of Nathaniel Trabotti, an Italian rabbi who died in 1658, as recorded by his disciple, Samuel Belgradi:

> He sanctified himself and said: Hear me, ye saints of the
> Lord! I am now 86 years of age, no more can I go and
> come in your midst as I have done from my early youth ...
> I have wronged none, but have tried my best to maintain
> union among you all small and great, so as to prevent
> scandals in your midst. Be gracious to me, my friends,
> and let your prayers be made on behalf of my soul, and I
> on my part will never cease to pray for you ... Many a
> time and oft, as I went about I heard the idle talk of
> gossiping women, who stood in the crossroads doing their
> work. They would croak like the frogs in Egypt while
> uttering the name of God and these doings were like
> needles in my flesh. I desired to suppress the fashion, but
> for various reasons was unable to translate thought into
> act. I do now order that any instance be reported
> forthwith to the rabbi and the latter shall prevent the
> continuance of the nuisance. Similarly I impose the same

rule against men who waste their time in gaming houses,
playing at dice and amusing themselves with cards,
which they always carry in their pockets. Let them desist
from their habit of using the Name of God in vain. Woe to
them, woe to their souls, woe to their latter end! I call
heaven and earth to witness that they must perish under
the dire wrath of God unless they mend their ways.[12]

He was certainly trying to control things beyond his own death, and many people continue to do that, as they think about their wills and how they will leave their money. The UK has no rules about how we divide up our assets for our survivors, but in France they do. When property is left, half has to go to the surviving partner and the rest to the children to be divided equally amongst them. This is part of the old Catholic view of equal division of property between surviving children, rather than the Protestant belief in keeping the property intact and leaving it to the eldest child, almost invariably the eldest son.

How we think about dividing up our property after our death may vary hugely between us, but one feature of growing older is that this becomes more and more important. We need a far greater debate about such things in the public domain. We are still reluctant to make our wills and to change them with changing circumstances. We are also disinclined to add a letter of intent to our heirs and executors about small bequests to friends and people we want to remember us well. These are important gifts and mementoes, and it is a shame that we do so little of it.

It is so easy to write a letter of intent and attach it to a will without going through the legal paraphernalia, and it is much appreciated. My mother was keen for all of her friends to have something to remember her by. She had many pictures of no great financial value, but they had fun – and we had fun – choosing something they would hang on their walls.

Another close friend of ours, Jim Rose, left many of his friends £250, and that was much appreciated. I used my money to buy a rather beautiful garden bench, and I think of him every time I see it. Similarly, my mother-in-law was keen that people she had known for many years, such as her hairdresser, should have something. My mother's housekeeper was delighted to have the silver tea set that my mother adored and used daily, and her housekeeper had cleaned weekly. I could list hundreds of other examples.

The point here, as we get older, is to realize that death will happen and that we have to prepare our wills. Everyone should have a will, however simple, and should take pleasure in adding to it the letter of intent that will allow them to give little things – a china ornament, a vase – to those they have loved and valued. This setting the scene, preparing the will and leaving the letter of intent, having the conversations with our children and relatives about what we want to happen and not happen, is so important.

It also gives a clue about some of the purpose of old age. It means allowing people the leisure to reflect on life as a whole, to run the film backwards, as the poem with which I began this book suggests. This reflection on our life, provided we could encourage it, and even sometimes formalize it, allows people to capture a sense of whether they have reached old age feeling satisfied, or the opposite. It gives people the space to consider using the last bit of their active lives to do some of the things they regret not having done, or to achieve goals they still haven't managed.

That approach, with a measured view of life as a whole, might lead to a different way of seeing old age, warts and all. It might lead to fantasies – an idealized old age, the granny contentedly knitting by the fire, minding the grandchild, with the cat purring at her feet.

It might also bring out people's worst fears about growing old. But at least it would be reflective, allowing people to think about being old, and thinking about what their life might have meant.

Good dying

Thanks to the hospice movement and our ability to control pain, we should be able to move away from fearing death itself. Most people are now convinced that hospices – both the institutions and the movement – can deal with the pain of dying, which is why the movement has become of one of Britain's great success stories, an export in thinking, intellectual and social, that has influenced care of the dying worldwide.

Hospices as we understand them started in the 1960s with a British woman, Cicely Saunders. A former nurse and medical social worker, she was appalled by the pain she saw amongst dying patients. She trained as a doctor, worked at St Joseph's Hospice in Hackney in East London, which is famous for having Irish Catholics down one side of the ward and orthodox Jews down the other, just because of the nature of the area. Miraculously, they have all always got on absolutely fine, with totally different attitudes to pain and to the end of life.

It is a hospice set up by the Irish order of the Sisters of Charity, who can really take the credit for the beginnings of the idea, but not its development into a total philosophy. When Cicely Saunders was there, despite the fact that everybody was getting on well, she was appalled by the lack of really serious pain control. She tried to improve it and to increase the doses of morphine. Finally, convinced that we needed to think differently, and by then a practising Christian, she resolved to open her own hospice.

She had been left £500 by one of her patients earlier in her career at St Thomas' Hospital, a young man called David Tasma, a Jewish refugee from the Warsaw Ghetto. He left it to her to be 'a window in your home'. By sheer force of personality, using that £500, she persuaded three major foundations to fund her hospice, and she opened St Christopher's Hospice in south-east London in 1967. She had, by then, established her definition of 'total pain' to be addressed by hospice care: 'physical, emotional, social or spiritual'. The World Health Organization still uses that definition, as do all the best textbooks.

The problem is that most of us don't die cared for by hospice teams or in hospices at all. In 2006, the *British Medical Journal* published a review of what is actually going on around people's deaths, which found that well over half of people with progressive illness want to die at home.[13] Despite this, most people in the UK, the USA, Germany, Switzerland and France die in hospitals. In the UK, the proportion of home deaths for patients with cancer is actually falling. Even the hospice movement is hugely geared to people with cancer, Motor Neurone Disease and AIDS, when most of us will die of something different.

In the UK, palliative care teams vary from place to place. Some offer care 24 hours a day, seven days a week, some just nine to five, five days a week. Pain control is often still appalling, and particularly so if cancer is not the condition concerned. That leaves us with a problem: how can we die well in a society which devotes most of its health care – resources, people and money – to hi-tech care and cure? And how can we reinvigorate the idea of total pain – physical, spiritual, social and emotional – when your average acute hospital wouldn't understand it, let alone be able to engage with it?

One of the most shocking facts about hospital care of older people, as we saw in the last chapter, is how many older people leave hospital malnourished and dehydrated. In fact, the failure to give food and drink may sometimes be in order to speed up the process of death. This is so different from what goes on when someone is actually dying, and they stop eating and drinking as their appetites shut down. Indeed, as Rabbi Jonathan Wittenberg put it elegantly in an article in the *Jewish Chronicle*, you can hear a family talk about a dying person and know what is going on.[14] They plead with their dying relative, 'Eat this!' (code for 'Come back!') and they tell you, 'Yesterday he managed a biscuit' (code for 'He's not dying ...').

The decision to stop feeding or giving liquids is significant. It shifts control from the dying person to the professional carers who, by their actions, are attempting to decide the time of death. There is a real question about deciding to stop giving ordinary food and liquids to very old people, in a society where many fail to understand the nature of artificial feeding by a plug in the stomach. Even so, older people are often not being fed and watered, and so they are not dying when, where and how they want. Who feeds, who eats, who drinks have become powerful moral questions.

When you look at the treatment of the very old at the time of dying, we tend to be kinder. That is why Muriel Gillick, in *The Denial of Ageing*, compared the speedy, natural deaths of centenarians with the uncomfortable, slow deaths of those who are younger at the hands of those who are determined 'officiously to keep alive'.[15]

In the hospices, managing total pain, and in assisted living facilities and nursing homes, day by day, you can see older people being given kind and good care. But it is not always true in other places, and that is why the debate about euthanasia has become so central and why movements for Physician Assisted Suicide are growing. Oregon already has this, though the numbers exercising it – 42 out of 30,000 deaths in 2004, if the data are to be believed – are tiny. In the UK, it has been debated time and again over the last few years in Parliament. In Switzerland, assisted suicide already exists with people travelling from all over Europe to access the clinic run by

Ludwig Minelli in Zürich. Belgium and the Netherlands have both euthanasia and Physician Assisted Suicide.

Whatever we may think about the morality of this, the debate is changing – and that is, at least in part, because people don't want intubated deaths in Intensive Care. They want to die at home, they want to be in charge and – for some reason – we don't want to let them. Hence the enthusiasm for something more extreme.

Across the world, we are seeing more and more disquiet about how we die. Even governments recognize it. So as concerned citizens we should be doing something to enable our fellow citizens and ourselves to die well when the time comes. There are three separate approaches we could adopt, which have some intellectual and ethical coherence, and we can all be involved in them.

Patient autonomy

We need to launch a debate about the nature of control, without it being diverted by the dispute, growing in anger and intensity, between those who have religious faith and the militant atheists, such as Richard Dawkins. We could try to establish that patient autonomy, a key principle in medical ethics, means being allowed to die where and how we want. That would mean that the system would simply have to change. It might not necessarily imply Physician Assisted Suicide, but it does mean being allowed to die well of whatever we are dying of.

Teach medical staff

There are many distinguished medical schools and nursing schools around the world, increasingly sharing syllabuses and exchanging teachers, and we need to press the authorities to make end-of-life care compulsory for all medical and nursing students. When we give 'the physician his place', as the Book of Ecclesiasticus in the Apocrypha tells us to do, that would mean they would have the knowledge, the skills and the understanding to be able to care for us better, and stop aggressive care earlier.

Define a good death

This is really the hardest question. We might recognize a good death when we see one, but still not be able to agree on a definition. Age Concern published some principles back in 2000 for their Millennium Debate of the Age.[16] Mostly they still stand, and the British Geriatric Society has signed up to them. They say that we should:

- be able to know when death is coming and understand what can be expected
- be able to retain control of what happens
- be afforded dignity and privacy
- have control over pain relief and other symptoms
- have choice and control over where death occurs
- have access to any spiritual and emotional support required
- have access to information and expertise of whatever kind is necessary
- have access to hospice care in any location, not only in hospital
- have control over who is present and who shares the end
- be able to issue advance directives which make sure wishes are respected
- have time to say goodbye and control over other aspects of timing

- be able to leave when it is time to go and not have life prolonged pointlessly.

If we could formulate some principles, those or others that we could all share – by all faiths, and all ethnic groups – it could really change the way we are treated. If we could do it so that spiritual pain is recognized as much as physical pain, so that getting ready to die well was seen as important, it might truly be transformational.

Scientists are saying most of us will get an additional 15 to 20 years of life. The question is whether we can use those extra years to take dying seriously, and capture all the great initiatives that have taken place around the world in hospice and palliative care, so the way we eventually die is universally good and the control is in our hands.

If we don't manage that, the danger is that euthanasia will be so much easier than helping people die well. It is cheaper than treating older people for depression, after all. It is administratively more straightforward than organizing hospice care. The danger is that, once we have it on the statute books, it will become decreasingly voluntary as the authorities reap the benefits, and then we will have even less control than before.

Call to arms

One of the great privileges I had whilst in the USA in 2006 was meeting the great writer and *bon vivant* Art Buchwald, in his hospice in Washington. He died, sadly, in early 2007, after a remission that was far longer than expected. He had written, broadcast and spoken of his impending death. He had no fear. His humour remained unabated. But as he looked you in the eye, he said some immensely serious things. First, that he was constantly learning even as he faced his own death. Second, that he was thinking about things people don't normally think about – such as the meaning of life and death. And third, that you need to think about the end of your life, whatever your life is.

This is a man who asked his friends to put an extra chair for him at the Seder table at Passover in April 2006. Not Elijah's chair as it would normally be, but Art's chair. In Jewish legend, Elijah the prophet will eventually sort out all the problems the rabbis couldn't solve. Elijah's place at Passover may exist because the rabbis never could decide quite how many cups of wine we had to drink, though we tend to drink four, with Elijah having a cup of his own that's usually untouched. In spring 2006 it was Art's chair, for Art's friends, as well as Elijah's.

The point was that Art was solving the problems and difficulties, and he was doing it by talking about what is unspeakable, by doing away with aggressive care, and by thinking and talking openly about his impending death. He wasn't in pain. His physical, social, emotional and spiritual pain were all being addressed. But he was saying that we all need to start thinking this way.

Dying like that – with our eyes open and without pain – means that we need not feel the guilt that goes with having a terrible end. Then, as we grieve for those who have lived a good long life and have died well, we will be able to let our tears fall naturally. 'My child,' says Ben Sirach, 'let your tears fall for the dead.' But perhaps not until we have completely changed the way many of the living are treated at the end of their lives.

So that is what the manifesto has to demand. **The medical profession must adopt a duty to allow people a good death, where they can be pain-free and in some control over how and where they die, and who they want to be there.**

This manifesto for old age is partly a manifesto for 'a good death' at the end of our days, something that was invented in the UK in the modern hospice movement, but seems sadly under threat as home deaths decrease, and as pressure mounts for euthanasia rather than dying well. It requires a new health infrastructure, better and more available palliative care, and more institutions like hospices, and a better understanding of the meaning, the stages and the moral demands of death among those who oversee it. But I believe we can do it.

The manifesto also needs to include demands to:

- **Make palliative care available whatever people are dying of and wherever they are dying, including nursing homes and care homes.** When I was a rabbinic student, we were taught a course called 'practical rabbinics', taught alternately by rabbis Lionel Blue and Hugo Gryn. Hugo organized for us all to go to St Christopher's hospice. Most of my fellow students really didn't want to go and I ended up going on my own, and it was an extraordinary experience. I found the way that people were talking quite compelling, out of a religious commitment – though it need not be religious – about giving people the space to die, which is partly about getting rid of the pain so it doesn't overwhelm you. Ever since, I have been furious that this space is only available in this country to people with cancer, when most people don't die of cancer.

  Both my parents were given excellent palliative care because they lived in a borough where it was available. If they had lived a few streets away across the borough boundary, they wouldn't have been given it. Of course, there should be local variations, but why have we accepted that people shouldn't be given palliative care in some places?

- **Give people the right to choose to die at home if they want to, and if it is possible.** The fact that the number of people dying in hospital is going up rather than down is a crying disgrace. It is also a false economy: hiding death away from relatives and society is bad for our mental health and entrenches the way society treats older people even further out of sight and out of mind.

- **Teach children about dying and make it visible.** Among the heroes of this chapter are the GPs who spend time with patients talking and reassuring them and their families about the process of dying. The best GPs are truly remarkable people and we should use them as community teachers as well, especially to children.

Chapter 10

Don't assume I'm not enjoying life, give me a chance

Grey rage

Why anyone wants to travel or study or go bungee jumping when they've got grandchildren is a mystery to me ... Never balk at being called 'granny'. It's not a dirty word, even though a friend of mine insists on being called 'Glammy'. It's a badge of honour, even when, like me, you're called Gaga.

Virginia Ironside, *How to Grow Old Disgracefully*

One of the tasks of later life, more especially for the years of retirement, is to look back at the joys and sorrows, the successes and failures, the unresolved problems and unfinished tasks of the past: to look back in order to let go.

Archbishop Robert Runcie, quoted in Shirley Toulson's book *The Country of Old Age*

We had a lovely friend in Ireland, a retired builder called Willy King, and I went to see him when he was dying. He was very clear and open about what was happening to him, but it was particularly lovely to see his great-granddaughter sitting on the bed playing with him as he told me about it.

When he was very near the end, the family brought his bed down to the kitchen and he lay there, with everybody else around – and all the coming and going – a part of everything that was going on. He wasn't pushed away anywhere to get on with it and his great-grandchildren and grandchildren were there with him. And I thought: why don't we all do that?

It is important that we should do so, partly because it is saner and very much better for the person who is dying. Partly also because it is saner and better for their relatives and helps with the grieving process. But partly also, and most importantly perhaps, because it will reduce people's fears of death, and I have become convinced that it is partly our fear of death – and our fears therefore of having to confront older people – that is driving their miserable treatment. We want them out of the way because we can't bear it; we are prepared to allow the cruellest and most degrading treatment because we feel safer when we don't contemplate old age at all.

If we can make people a little less frightened, then we will have more chance of putting this manifesto into practice. In this, as in so many other areas, older people may have to be the agents of change themselves. What is exciting is that, perhaps for the first time in human history, they are also increasingly able to do this. All around us, older people are waking up and taking back their lives.

This is an angry book, and it made me angry to research it. But it is a contrasting picture as well, because I found myself wanting to shout about the hope as well as the hell of it. Amongst the gloom of poor care, there is terrific care going on. Amongst the bad health, there is amazing health. Amongst the frailty, there is terrific spirit. Time and again, older people are refusing to play to the media picture of them at all.

Coming alive in old age

I went to London's Capital Age Festival in Coin Street in August 2006, which asked people to: 'Be a wild child and let your hair down'. With a mixture of tea tent and the Blackfriars Reminiscence Project, there were interactive performances, classic Indian dancing, hand and nail massage, and people getting their cholesterol, blood pressure and sugar levels tested. There was jiving and Latin American dance, the South African Proteas, Jackie and Rose with Cuban dancing, and so on. This whole festival was – and is – an expression of joy at being alive.

But it isn't just festivals. Old people, like everyone else, like a bit of a risk, or just being plain stroppy. There was Gwen Dorling, 102, who told workers at her care home in Diss in Norfolk that she would have liked a male stripper for her hundredth birthday.[1] So she got one for her 102nd birthday instead, and has asked for two for her 103rd.

There was the great-grandmother, 85, who was fighting to be able to strip off and sunbathe topless in her garden after permission was granted for 43 new houses and flats behind her bungalow in Fareham, Hampshire. 'It's just absurd,' she said. 'Why should I have to stop taking my clothes off to sunbathe because a developer wants to build something so high with windows facing us? I need to strip off and I don't think people should be looking at me ... There's a lot of elderly people along here who sunbathe. Why should we have to stop because of some overpriced flats?'[2]

There was Rose Hacker, who died aged 101 and had been a weekly columnist on the *Camden New Journal* till the time of her death. She embodied the spirit of the good life for old people. She was an accomplished sculptor, took up T'ai Chi in her 80s, and was a lifelong pacifist and socialist. A relationship counsellor and author of bestselling books on teenage sex, she lived her last years at the Mary Fielding Trust, and had her stage début, with two fellow residents, dancing in something specially choreographed for them at the age of 101. She also took on officialdom to the end. Dame Denise Platt, chair of the Commission for Social Care Inspection, shared a platform with her a couple of months before she died, and was told afterwards: 'Denise, I am not a tick box. I am more than a tick box, I am a person.'[3]

There was even the man who stole vegetables off other people's allotments. Philip Powner, 76, became the first person to be banned from setting foot in any allotment or garden under an antisocial behaviour order.[4] He isn't even the oldest person with an Asbo, who is actually 88. Germany is building three new prisons for older people: in 2005, the notorious 'Grandpa gang' – a trio of pensioners aged between 64 and 74 – were found guilty of robbing 14 banks over 16 years and sentenced to a total of 31 years in jail.[5]

Then there are The Zimmers, the rock group featured in Chapter 5. The American based Young@heart chorus goes from success to success, touring the world. The Rolling Stones roll on in their sixties, though the over-45s were banned from one of their concerts in 2006. Older women give birth, despite widespread disapproval, including Rosanna Della Corte, 62. There was even the wonderful story of older drivers who are more 'mischievous' with satnav, when three quarters of over-50s deliberately use different routes to confuse their satellite equipment. A third of men and a fifth of women over 80 use mobile phones.

Community Care magazine found that older people are no longer afraid to tell day centres and nursing homes what they want. Marion Bulkan, an entertainment organizer at a London day centre, says that service users are ever more sophisticated: 'Our entertainment has to be of a professional standard.' She organizes four shows a week for an audience partial to a bit of Robbie Williams, Sinatra and Elvis. 'If they like it, they join in ... If they don't, they start talking or just walk out.'[6]

Older people are talking more openly about sex, and looking for new partners after divorce or bereavement. They always did, but the ONS shows more over-50s getting divorced than ever before. 'Years ago when people got into their fifties, they'd start thinking it was pipe and slipper time,' says Paula Hall of relationship counsellors Relate. 'But increasingly, longevity means they have more time up their sleeves now, and they're thinking more about what they really want to do with that time.'[7]

Even people with Alzheimer's are shifting the way we look at them. Julie Christie's magnificent performance in the film *Away from Her* showed how a woman with Alzheimer's forms an emotional attachment to another man in her care home, to her husband's deep distress and eventual acceptance. There was also the story of former Supreme Court Justice Sandra Day O'Connor's husband, who also has Alzheimer's and formed an attachment to another woman in a care home. The former justice said that it was a relief to see her husband of 55 years so content.[8]

An American survey has demonstrated that sex looms large in the lives of the over-60s, with a high proportion of men and women remaining intimately active well into old age.[9] There is some similar evidence for the UK from a much smaller study. So it's a mixed picture, and clearly sexual activity is going on longer than people had previously thought. Maybe it always has, but the public imagination could not face the fact. Or maybe the fact we are living longer means that all our appetites continue longer. Whichever is the case, it is clear that policy makers for care homes, or any kind of housing development, have to accept that sex and intimacy are here to stay for older people, whatever anyone else thinks.

Given that, there is a great deal of online dating for the over-50s, with women being three quarters of the users, and women complaining that it is much harder to find a partner once they have turned 60. Yet keeping trying seems important, and people do. The columnist Virginia Ironside's witty look at sex in later life for women claimed that 'there is a big fashion for anyone over 60 to claim that they have just as much sex as they ever did'.[10]

'Really? Really, really, really?' she asked. 'Most women, when I mention sex, wince in agony at the thought of it. Although it's taboo to say it, sex for an enormous number of women after the menopause simply gets more and more agonizing ... No sex means you can flirt much, much more without the risk of it all going too far ... and if, occasionally, you do have sex, well, what a treat. Even if you have to live on cranberry juice for two months afterwards.'

Virginia Ironside's slightly acerbic approach also tackles the issue of making friends:

> By the time you're 60, your address book (that is, if you
> keep one, which if you're like me you do, dreading risking
> them being stored in an iPod that might crash at any
> time) gets to be huge, and your writing tinier and tinier.

That means some names have to go. It is true that I have friends who do a cull of the address book every ten years. Reading Ironside, it sounds like it will need to be every five years or less after 60. Not only address books either, because, as Ironside explains, our confidence improves with age. 'It means you dare ask people to explain if you don't understand what they're saying,' she writes, 'that you can burst into wreaths of smiles at strangers in the street (much, often, to their consternation, but who cares about that) and that when you order a rare steak in a restaurant and you're brought a piece of leather, you have no compunction in, very kindly and sweetly, sending it back.'[11]

She is right. Older age does bring a kind of confidence. We care less about the impression we make, about making a fuss or admitting we don't understand. This is new: the previous generation of older people didn't have that confidence, and we should celebrate the newfound assertiveness of older people, and their ability get what they want, and say no. If they could only manage it in a care situation, it would make for a great old age for all of us.

Reflection

What with the recently published reflections on age by Virginia Ironside, and people like the publisher Diana Athill and the journalist Katherine Whitehorn, there seems to be another important shift going on. It is now fashionable to reflect on this stage of life, and this suggests we are beginning to rouse ourselves to look clearly at old age again. The fact that we want to hear people's own reflections on facing their own mortality might be an opportunity to do something to help all those people who won't be able to do that, even privately.

'In old age we are reaping the fruits: not a sudden lurch into a smelly decline, but vistas of years ahead of modest pleasures,' writes Joan Bakewell.[12] 'Horizons that are no longer set by the needs of family, the career ambitions, the immediate and intense business of daily survival.' She describes the enthusiasms, the University of the Third Age, the Open University, the travels, the mountain climbing, the sponsored walks and climbs for charity. She adds that one friend in his late seventies 'has recently taken up tap dancing. How's that for bravura!'

She also asks for a change in the way we think about retirement: 'There must be more varied and adaptable options than simply working full tilt till 60 then slamming the door on all your wisdom and experience. We shall all certainly have to work longer ... but that doesn't mean we have to stay in the rat ace, with the stress and the competitive thrust that gives middle age its ulcers.'

Joan Bakewell's volume of short essays started life as a series of columns for the *Guardian*, entitled 'Just Seventy'. Moving and wise, they were wonderful to read, and it is a source of great sadness to many of us, younger and older, that she hasn't continued writing them. She wrote them to make herself feel valued, that she still 'belonged to the community of journalists among whom I had worked for many decades'. Of course she could carry on working after 70, and she does, just as that famous veteran warhorse of a journalist, Bill Deedes, died in journalistic harness at 94 in August 2007, having seen his own son retire before him.

Joan Bakewell reflects on faith, too. She expected, as that whole generation did, that religion would have died out, yet it is stronger than ever. She still goes to carol services, often as fundraisers for good causes. The one she reflects on most sombrely was the St Martin in the Fields service expressing support for the Guantanamo Bay Human Rights Commission in their efforts 'to right one of the world's most conspicuous wrongs'.

Joan Bakewell has always been interested in issues of faith, and has presented many faith programmes. But other older people are being more quizzical about faith, including Shirley Toulson, in her moving book *The Country of Old Age*, one of the best attempts to write about how ageing feels, in spiritual and other terms. She quotes Etty Hillesum, the young Dutch Jew who perished in the Nazi concentration camps, as defining the task that confronts us all to our dying day as a determination to 'find out how to come to terms with our bad moods without making others suffer from them':

> *We have just one moral duty: to reclaim large areas of peace in ourselves, more and more peace, and reflect it towards others. And the more peace there is in us, the more peace there will be in our troubled world.*[13]

Shirley Toulson also wrote about how to look back on the past:

> *The garden of the past has to be carefully cultivated or it will infect my future in all sorts of ways. Above all, it is essential that I forgive the past, both for the ways in which I may feel that I have been victimized by it and for my own part in smirching it. The paradox is that until I determine to leave the past I cannot truly forgive it, yet the only way to forgive the past is to look at it from my present viewpoint.*[14]

She also quotes Charles Williams, the colleague of Tolkien and C. S. Lewis, when he described the feelings of the dying nonagenarian Margaret Anstruther as being 'absent not with the senility of a spirit wandering in feeble memories, but with the attention of a worker engrossed'.[15]

The Royal College of Psychiatrists has become more interested in these issues too, with a joint conference held by its Faculty of Old Age Psychiatry and its Spirituality and Psychiatry special interest group in 2005, at which Andrew Powell presented a paper which looks at how patients hold up to their doctors a mirror which makes them realize there is no difference between patient and doctor – and that the relationship is what can bring help, for whether one believes in God or not 'the spiritual impulse makes itself known just the same'.[16]

All these are attempts to come to some description of the spiritual awareness many older people have. Attendances at places of worship are, on the whole, overwhelmingly of older people. Older people find comfort, familiarity, music and community in their churches, mosques and synagogues. But this spirituality is something less formal. It echoes Milton's 'all passion spent'. It describes a way of looking back in calm, but working at it, and knowing that old age is a journey that is also a spiritual journey.

It is a time when people describe huge energy, often difficult to use properly, when they think great thoughts and write them down, and when the greatest artists paint old age in a golden light, as Rembrandt did in his later self-portraits.

None of this is a bed of roses. Despite all this possibility and time, old age remains – as Mary Riddell put it in the *Observer* –'such a barren place'.[17] 'You feel like surprised leftovers, in shrinking time and fading light,' wrote Richard Hoggart.[18] The artist Goya looked unflinchingly at old age in his last works.[19] His drawings included twisted faces, knotty bone, stooped porters, or the madman with a single eye swivelling in his skull. But we can learn from his ability to look at age, and the rest of our lives, unflinchingly and in the round, with all the possibilities and horrors together.

If we can do that, and help our children do it, if we can roll back that fear of old age that does so much damage – and the fear of death that lies behind it – then we can find the will as a society to put the manifesto into effect. Without it, the fear will take over, and we will be left with rising demands for euthanasia, knowing that – as in Holland and other places – once enacted, it tends to become less voluntary.

The euthanasia debate and the fear of old age go hand in hand. People feel that old age is pointless time, that older people are unnecessary, and they don't want to be like that themselves. I don't have a principled objection to people committing suicide in some circumstances, if they can square it with those who love them. But I do object to them expecting other people to kill them, especially as it will encourage our rulers to forget about the quality of care. Why worry about it, after all, if you can just shoot old people?

Of course there will always be exceptional and difficult cases. But simple loss of control is not a good enough reason, it seems to me, to expect doctors to take lives. Life isn't about being in control: we have no control as babies and sometimes we must face losing control as we get older too. Once again, we have to look at it squarely in the face – and the final loss of control in death as well. Then we can calm people's fears and avoid the non-solution of euthanasia.

Politics

But simply calming people's fears isn't enough to confront the sheer injustice. We need political will, and that needs to come from older people themselves. They are now more important as voters. Over-55s accounted for 41 per cent of votes cast at the 2005 general election (compared with 37 per cent for 18–24s). Age Concern is tracking constituencies which will have older voter majorities by 2009, so governments are more likely to listen – especially with 17 million baby boomers heading towards retirement. Yet they still threw out the EU directive to stop employers forcing people to retire at state pension age if they had the skills and capacity to continue.

There is political progress. The Link Age Plus programme is being piloted in eight local authority areas across England, from Devon to Tyne and Wear, with older people getting the right to shape their own health and social care services. This is the Sure Start model, and is really important. Discrimination in some areas is being outlawed, from car insurance to the workplace. Ireland has begun a serous Age Equality programme, launched with a flourish in 2007. The Irish Equality Authority took on the car rental and car insurance providers over blanket bans on age grounds. Sally Greengross, former chef executive of Age Concern and now of the International Longevity Centre, has managed to highlight discrimination in insurance, car hire, borrowing money and healthcare, as well as the assumptions on slowing up in learning and acquiring skills.[20]

But still I wish they would punch harder, and not let government off the hook when it fails to stop the CBI objecting to getting rid of a mandatory retirement age. The problem is that politicians still don't listen to the views of older people when they make decisions.

'I've lived and worked in Southwark for more years than I like to think and I don't think it's just Southwark – I think most councils are the same,' said one older person quoted in Help the Aged's 2007 report *Social Inclusion and Older People – A Call for Action.*[21] 'It doesn't matter if they're Labour or Liberal. I just said to my husband this morning: "What is it? Where do they get these people? Where do these people come from who don't live here, who've got a job?" They sit and look at the people and they treat them with contempt. What sort of people are they – do they not care about anything, about us, about the community? They've got no feeling, they've not got parents, they've not got children ... They've got no right. It's not fair.'

This kind of anger is relatively new, and it is changing things a little. Politicians are learning they have to listen to older people's views, even though their political induction, some years ago, would have conditioned them not to bother to do so. What was so heart-warming about most older people I met and talked to while I was researching this book was that they were all worth listening to, and deserved to be listened to as of right. It isn't instrumental. It isn't just to make services better – it's because they have something to say, and we should listen. What they have to say might also help us create a better society, but that is almost beside the point.

There are some lively signs around, if somewhat few and far between. The North Staffordshire Pensioners' Convention made a protest film to show WH Smith managers in Stoke on Trent in July 2007, to try to persuade them that moving the post office from Hanley to the branch of Smiths in the Potteries shopping centre was a bad idea for older people, who would find it more difficult to get to.[22] Then there is Josephine Rooney, the redoubtable campaigner from Derby, who was jailed at the age of 69 for three months for refusing to pay her council tax in protest at the crime-filled street in which she lived, dubbed 'crack alley' because of the drug users who meet there.[23] And the direct action activist Irene Willis, 'who knew she was not cut out for the stereotypical pensioner's life when she retired', and has been chaining herself to fences and breaking into nuclear bases, and getting herself imprisoned for a few days at a time for refusing to pay fines.[24] 'When you get old, suddenly no one listens to you any more,' she says. 'Direct action makes you feel empowered ... I can afford to go to prison – I'm not going to lose my job; I'm not going to lose my house.' There are also the substantial numbers of council tax protesters back in 2005 who were virtually queuing up to go to jail, with retired vicar Alfred Ridley, 71, and former social worker, Sylvia Hardy, 73, being only the first.

Even so, the political anger required to make real change happen still isn't there. Only Raymond Tallis, former professor of geriatric medicine, really comes out with a call to the barricades. He argues that it is to older people themselves that we should be looking for criticism of the status quo:

> *Where, then, are we to look for the guardians of freedom? This is where the growing cadre of healthy elderly people may be increasingly important. They no longer yearn for promotion or preferment. They aren't required to bite their tongue or grovel. They have no targets to deliver on, no need to devote themselves to the futile productivity of academe, no asinine mission statements to write or respond to. They are at liberty to think and say what they like. They can therefore shout out what those who have families to feed or careers to promote – and so must remain on message at all costs – would not dare mutter in their sleep. Because they have nothing to lose by speaking the truth ... they are ... a precious resource that we can ill afford to overlook ... This is not an argument for a cognitive gerontocracy but a call for this new and growing generation of rentiers to take up the battle to defend the freedoms they have enjoyed but which, if present trends are unopposed, their grandchildren may not.*[25]

Professor Tallis is absolutely right, but it is not just about freedoms, but also about opportunities. Nor are we there yet. We have yet to see the determination for change, and that's what we want. Not 'Isn't she marvellous?' nor 'What a shame, she'd be better off dead.' No barren places or isolation, no praise for age alone, but something much more coherent and furious. Hence writing this manifesto for old age. And if other people don't get on with it, I will be on the barricades myself.

We certainly need a real change on the part of the voluntary organizations that exist to represent older people. Because they are largely driven by their need to fundraise, they talk up the 'victimhood' of older people and deskill older people themselves – who begin to believe they do not have a voice. They have allowed the agenda to be set in a way that sets young against old, youth unemployment versus early retirement of older people to make room for the young, or health services where people feel they have had their day and must leave the resources to the young.

They have allowed those old assumptions to continue and it is time they focused on the isolation of older people, the purchasing power of the grey pound, the disgrace of malnutrition amongst older people when we have an epidemic of obesity amongst younger people, on the lack of access to psychological therapies for older people.

Because these big agencies are potentially in the front line of this battle, they could be instrumental in launching the grey panther movement, a powerful cross-party alliance of older people who have an interest in changing perceptions and practice, and will fight to get what they want. But while the charities stay fearful that they will lose their government funding, the movement may have to be launched by others.

Behind all that, there is a broad moral case to be made to wake society up. How can highly trained professionals like doctors and nurses accept such degrading treatment of older people, to the extent that older people are allowed to lie in their own excrement in hospitals or be told to 'go in your pants', as if that was acceptable for any of us? How have we trained them to turn a blind eye to this?

How have we managed to focus media attention solely on children who are abused, when the abuse of vulnerable older people is everywhere? We need a collective wake-up call to see what is staring us in the face.

Along with that wake-up call, we need to launch a series of debates on the nature and meaning of old age, on what families should take responsibility for – the idea that a family is not responsible for its own older members is deeply shocking, but we owe them support to take that responsibility – and about dying well, moving away from the arid euthanasia discussion to what kind of deaths we want, where and who we want with us.

Once we have that wake-up call, and the grey panthers to deliver it, what will they demand? This book has pieced together a manifesto for them. It isn't complete and much of it requires policy that still needs developing, but it falls into the following ten urgent categories:

1. End discrimination against people on the grounds of age

We must do this whether it is in healthcare, insurance, volunteering or the right to work. This has been allowed to continue in a way it is just inconceivable that others forms of discrimination would be allowed. This also means tackling the endemic ageism in the NHS and other institutions, which add up their Quality of Life Adjusted Years – the so-called QALYs that health planners use – and then apply them to individuals regardless of their needs, desires or conditions.

We have to insist that health professionals provide access to the services and treatments – especially for strokes and depression – that they need, that they ignore QALYs and focus on the individuals before them, insisting that they have a conversation with individuals and their families about their lives as they get older, to focus on what they feel is important, not what the policy says they should feel.

2. The right to work, so that older people who are capable of carrying out a useful working role should be allowed to do so, no matter how old they are

It is time to ban compulsory retirement ages, and we will need to do so if we are to get older people to use their skills beyond 60 or 65, as they will have to do if we are not going to face a crisis in pension income over the next generation. And if older people have the right to work, that should include a right to play a role in front-line politics without endless carping about their age, and a right to front TV programmes without television executives throwing up their hands in horror. That does not imply older people doing what they did when they were younger, but it does imply them working in some way – paid or voluntarily – in order to keep the mind active and to have a reason to get up in the morning. They will also need the education and training for the work and activities they are undertaking.

What applies to work also needs to apply to volunteering, especially if we are to get older volunteers in much bigger numbers to provide mutual support and to humanize public services for other older people. Volunteering will become a key part of even more older people's activity, but needs real effort injected into it to make it meaningful and satisfying. The Experience Corps has had a difficult time, as have some other volunteering endeavours for older people, despite the large numbers of older people volunteering. The government will need to think again about how to engage older people in volunteering in a less preachy, less bossy way, and to provide support for people to do it. It will also need to provide more consistent funding for the voluntary sector bodies that are there to reach out to older people and bring them into the unpaid workforce.

3. Integrate tax and pensions so that everyone gets what they are entitled to

It is insane that older people are expected to claim for a whole range of tiny pots of money to cover specific needs, so that those who are most in need are forced to be supplicants for hand-outs. Integrated tax and benefits means the government could calculate what they owed to people, minus tax, and provide the proper sum, without having the indignity of applying. We also need to end the link between our retirement age and the age when we draw our pension, and focus pension resources on those who really are beginning to be unable to work at all. The idea that we can retire at 65, 60 or even 55 is not sustainable, and probably never has been, and is giving rise to fears of a 'demographic time bomb', which in turn is fuelling resentment of the needs of older people and fear of them in society.

In the meantime, we need benefits offices to take responsibility for reaching out to vulnerable older people to make sure they get whatever benefits they are eligible for. Very large percentages of benefits are not taken up in old age, and this exacerbates poverty. Without this outreach system, the state is in fact discriminating against older people, because they know that they tend not to fight for their benefits. We also need a raft of more imaginative financial products aimed at ordinary people, which will allow them to save better for care needs, cash in the value of homes without undermining their eligibility for state support, and encourage them to get better after hospital visits – and go home again – rather than sinking into inexorable decline.

4. An elected standing committee of over-70s to hold every local authority to account

This committee should be able to compel any public official to answer questions and to write an annual report on the state of the area from an older people's point of view, which will go to the Audit Commission. They should have the power to question those responsible on specific issues like an American-style Grand Jury. And the first issue they need to tackle is to force councils to take responsibility for making sure there are enough public toilets in town centres, the absence of which is a major limit on the freedom of many older people. Plus seats in shops, park benches and park wardens – so that older people do not just give up, stay at home and become isolated. Older people need to reclaim the streets.

The committee needs to drive moves to bring in older people to monitor and help deliver council services. Our failure to do this so far means we are wasting the time and talents of older people. We also need to force developers to show they have worked with local groups of older people before any planning application is given approval.

It hardly needs saying that we also need to insist on effective public transport in rural areas to suit older people. People who are still working, whatever their age, should not be given a Freedom Pass, however popular it is; those who are not working, who live in areas with poor public transport and who no longer drive, need far greater attention. That means thinking through the implications of rural transport schemes for older people – and others without transport for whatever reason – often to be run by voluntary sector organizations or social enterprises, but paid for partly out of the public purse.

Apart from providing seating, shops will also need to be better at providing clothes for older people without making them feel distinctly unfashionable. Better fitting rooms, older sales staff and a better range of suitable clothes would all help. Fashion chains need to chase the grey pound, and older people should refuse to spend any money at all in stores where sales assistants are not unfailingly welcoming and polite.

5. Access for older people, at a reasonable cost, to whatever education will allow them to grow as people

Of course, it is also reasonable that they should have to pay, but it is counter-productive to expect older people on pensions to pay the full costs. Such a policy is more humane, more life-affirming, and also in the long run a good deal healthier – and therefore cheaper to the public purse – than a narrowing of education to its most youthful and utilitarian. The current emphasis on education and training for work purposes has its place, but it is short-sighted in the extreme to cut older people off from further and higher education by cost.

They may continue to work in the paid work marketplace, if things change over retirement ages, as seems likely. But even more important is the fact that many older people will contribute in other ways, through voluntary activity, to their communities, and cutting them off from education and training makes no sense.

Sports and leisure will need to be rethought too, and adapted to suit older people to a greater extent. Single-sex swimming is largely designed for some religious groups, but it suits older women very well, and needs to be expanded. Local authorities need to restrict some times for use of their facilities for older people, particularly those who are frailer, for whom keeping fit is of vital importance if they are going to avoid becoming housebound, and thereby an increasing charge on taxpayers.

6. Genuine choice in housing, including lifetime homes, communes, co-housing and other mutual housing solutions

It really is extraordinary that co-housing should be so difficult here. We need to re-invent housing associations, set them free from the straitjacket that forces them to hand over nomination rights to new homes to the local authority, and let them spin off experimental organizations that imaginative people can invest in, and allow them to find new solutions for staying put when people are older. It is a crying shame that housing for older people in the United States and in most of Europe is far superior to ours, and infinitely more imaginative. We also need to insist that a 'home for life' is just what it says. That means that sheltered housing has to extend to palliative care and proper care for people with dementia. It is time that older people were given a real choice about where they are to live.

We can certainly build houses and ground-floor flats so that they can be adapted easily for older people to provide them with genuinely lifetime homes, which can accommodate them until they die. Nor is there any reason why we can't provide sheltered housing, with nursing care, and co-housing options in every neighbourhood. Why should we expect older people to move away from everything and everyone familiar when they get older, when moving is most traumatic?

The other urgent need, to help older people stay put, is a reliable network of handyperson services which specialize in repair work for older people. Local authorities must also provide proper advice about housing options for older people. There is almost no comprehensive information available at the moment, either about what is available or about the costs involved.

7. Turn care into an honourable, trained, better-paid profession

Care workers will need to be both better trained and better paid. We need to end the way nurses treat care assistants as the ones who do the dirty jobs. They will probably have to form themselves into some kind of social enterprise model to provide local services, with administration provided for groups of them centrally.

Care services must also be reformed so that social services departments have far less say on how services are provided. Individual payments should become the norm unless the people who need the services are not mentally capable of doing the choosing and paying, where family members, volunteers or paid professional assistants will need to help. Older people who are frail should be able to choose how they want their services provided, and if they choose to spend more on getting out of the house – with however much difficulty – than on meals on wheels, that is their business.

We badly need a settlement around how much people should need to have to spend themselves on care, and what needs to be available for paying for care needs beyond that. The welcome hint in the government's comprehensive spending review in October 2007 that there might be a review of how long-term care is paid for, possibly based on the Wanless model, is one sign that some part of older people's campaigning has paid off. Attitudes to inheritance tax also need to be re-examined. Certainly older people are going to have to be willing to pay for their own long-term care up to a certain, agreed, point.

There also needs to be a change in local funding arrangements to encourage small, family-run care homes: at the moment these are discouraged by the way payments are made. The result is that homes are increasingly large, less human places, where relationships are even more difficult to build with staff and where rules are even more inflexible.

8. Rebuild an NHS network of convalescent beds and community hospitals

That is the best way of helping older people recover after hospital stays, and without which they are at the mercy of hospital administrators complaining about 'bed blockers', but the network will have to be bolstered by proper support at home and a new generation of mutual volunteer support. While there are still scandals like those at Maidstone and Pembury hospitals, with large numbers still dying from *clostridium difficile*, a cause of diarrhoea and sickness that particularly attacks older people, it is difficult to see the wood for the trees. Yet such scandals themselves should tell us that nursing standards have slipped abysmally if staff think it at all acceptable to leave patients in their own excrement. There can be no excuse, and it demonstrates an utter lack of consideration for the dignity of the patients in their care. So older people will need to ask tough questions of their local hospitals, and GPs will need to think twice about referring patients there while they remain dangerous, Dickensian places, moving back towards a nineteenth-century view that says people should be nursed at home as far as possible. That might require more night and weekend work from GPs and district nurses, but it might in the end be more satisfactory for everyone, as they will have happier, less distressed and demoralized patients.

Scandals apart, older people and their healthcare advisers will need to do some real thinking about what older people themselves want and need. There will need to be serious trade-offs made between local access and regional excellence, with many older people favouring the local. Not all sections of the population, even in the older population, will see this the same way, but part of the settlement is going to be this new network of local community hospitals, specializing in sensitive care for older people near their home, some even run by the voluntary sector.

There certainly needs to be an end to discrimination in healthcare. There will always have to be some kind of rationing in the NHS, but it is indefensible that this should be done on the basis of age, so that older people are always at the end of the queue, always get the cheapest solutions. Part of the answer is going to be changes in the way health professionals are trained, sending trainees to live with a family of someone with a long-term condition to get that personal perspective before the endemic ageism of the NHS creeps up on them.

9. The right to a good death, pain-free, and control over how and where it happens, and over who we want to be there

Everyone has the right to what the hospice movement has developed, including palliative care to give people the space to die well, no matter where they live and what they are dying of. That also means giving people the right to choose to die at home if they want to, and if it is possible. The fact that the number of people dying in hospital is going up rather than down is disgraceful. It is also a false economy to hide death away from relatives and society, and fuels the fear of death and age which in turn is driving the cruelty. We need to teach children about dying and make it visible.

10. Launch a grey panthers movement, get angry, force change to happen

There is some evidence, though not much, that older people are beginning to fight back and to realize the political power they potentially possess. But what we need now is to focus that anger, not just by expecting politicians and professionals to change – though they surely must – but by setting up the businesses, services, mutual networks and new designs for living that older people will need. Nobody is going to do this for them. What they have to realize is that they have the power, energy and time to make it happen for themselves.

That is a manifesto for the new movement, but it is also worth giving a short warning on false solutions – those ideas, often technological, that are pedalled as major solutions to ageing, but are actually tools to make it easier to maintain the current outrageous status quo. There is nothing wrong with the idea of watching your elderly mother, 200 miles away, through a video screen. It might provide early warning of accidents. But what it emphatically is not is a solution to her isolation. Quite the reverse. Nor are other technological systems that monitor older people at home but never provide them with human contact.

In the same way, you have to be sceptical about the government's solution of 'polyclinics' – large GP surgeries designed to cope with bigger demands – when it is precisely the individual relationships with GPs which policy-makers are discounting that make such a difference to older people's lives.

Nor, of course, is euthanasia – all these are solutions which assuage the guilt of those who run the systems, and let people off the hook while further isolating older people. They have their place in a battery of ideas, but they are not solutions.

At the heart of everything is the need to shift people's attitudes to old age, but that will happen as a result of the manifesto. It isn't a necessary condition. Much of this shift would be easier if we stopped regarding successful and remarkable older people as exceptional, and instead accepted them as the norm – PhD students, rock groups, criminals and exercise fanatics alike. Only then would it be possible to say that experience is as valuable as the freshness of youth, just different. Stigmatizing older people by making them pay for what younger people get free is wrong – even if they can afford it, as in the case of further education.

Only then could we argue that stability, as manifested in older people's lives, is valuable just as change is inevitable, and that the two are in a healthy tension, but with neither preferable to the other. Only then will we be able to recognize the wisdom age brings, the capacity to see the wood for the trees, the recognition of investing for children and grandchildren, that makes a society feel at ease with itself.

But if we fail to rethink our attitude to older people in the UK, I believe we will head even faster towards a fractured society in which various groups, older people included, will feel they have no part, and no care for the future. And that would be a disaster.

Notes

Introduction

1   *The Guardian* (2006), 4 Jan.
2   King's Fund (2001), *Future Imperfect?*

Chapter 1

1   House of Lords Science and Technology Committee (2005), *Ageing: Scientific Aspects.*
2   Jill Sherman (2007), 'Wealthy, healthy, and aged 85: the woman living ever longer', *Times*, 25 Oct.
3   *Daily Mail* (2006), 8 Feb.
4   *Guardian* (2006), 8 Feb.
5   Ibid.
6   Geraldine Bedell (2005), 'The third agers', *Observer*, 30 Oct.
7   Stephen Moss (2006), 'Life at 100', *Guardian*, 18 Jan.
8   Ibid.
9   Mary Riddell (2006), 'Longer lifespans are a bit of a grey area', *Observer*, 12 Feb.
10 Ibid.
11 Diana Athill (2007), *Somewhere Towards the End*, London, p. 125.
12 A.Bowling and P. Dieppe (2005), 'What is successful ageing and who should define it?', *BMJ*, 331: pp. 1548–51 (24 Dec).

13 J.W. Rowe and R.L. Kahn (1998), *Successful Ageing*, New York, Pantheon Books.

14 W.J. Strawbridge, M.L. Wallhagen and R.D. Cohen (2002), 'Successful ageing and wellbeing: Self-rated compared with Rowe and Kahn', *Gerontologist*, 42: pp. 727–32.

15 Christopher Callahan and Colleen McHorney (2003), 'Successful ageing and the humility of perspective', *Annals of Internal Medicine*, 2 Sept, vol 139, pp. 389–90.

16 A.Bowling and P. Dieppe (2005), 'What is successful ageing and who should define it?', *BMJ*, 331: pp. 1548–1551 (24 Dec).

17 Katharine Whitehorn (2007), *Selective Memory*, London, pp. 262–3.

18 Muriel Gillick (2006), *The Denial of Ageing: Perpetual Youth, Eternal Life, and Other Dangerous Fantasies*, Harvard University Press, Cambridge, Massachusetts and London, pp. 213–4.

19 *Times* (2005), 6 Aug.

20 Diana M. Jelley (2006), 'Which patients with which needs are leading the patient led NHS?', *BMJ*, 332; p. 1221 (20 May).

Chapter 2

1 Joan Bakewell (2006), 'What I see in the mirror', *Guardian*, 7 Oct.

2 Diana Athill (2007), *Somewhere Towards the End*, Granta, London, p. 15.

3 Michele Hanson (2006), 'Ladies – let yourselves go!', *Guardian*, 30 Aug.

4 Virginia Ironside (2007), *No, I Don't Want to Join a Book Club*, Penguin, London.

5   Age Concern discussion forums (2005): Should I dress and
    live like the age I'm supposed to be?
    http://www.ageconcern.org.uk/discuss/index.cm
6   *Independent* (2006), 29 Apr.
7   Hamish McRae (2005), 'Pension reform is one thing –
    persuading us to work longer is another', *Independent,* 1 Dec.
8   *Observer* (2006), 12 Feb.
9   Social Exclusion Unit: Older people and employment web
    page.
10 Roberston, I., Warr., P., Butcher, V., Callinan, M. & Bardzill, P.,
    (2002) *Older People's Experience of Paid Employment:
    Participation and Quality of Life.* ESRC Growing Older
    Programme Research Findings no. 14.
11 Joseph Rowntree Foundation (2003), *The Role of Flexible
    Employment for Older Workers*, York.
12 Doyal, L. and Payne, S. (2006), *Older Women, Work and Health:
    Reviewing the Evidence*, Help the Aged and TAEN (The Ageing
    and Employment Network), London.
13 James Harding (2007), 'UK plc is undervaluing age and
    experience', *Times*, 1 Jun.
14 Janet Street-Porter (2005), 'Our ageist attitudes have got to
    change', *Independent,* 8 Sep.
15 *Times Online* (2006), 8 Feb.
16 Sally Price (2007), *Volunteering in the Third Age: Final Report*,
    VITA, London.
17 *Age Shall Not Weary Them Nor the Years Condemn: Retired
    and Senior Volunteering Today,* WRVS and CSV (2006)
18 Ibid.
19 WRVS (2007), Press pack for WiseLine launch, Nov.
20 Colin Rochester and Thomas, Brian (2006), *The Indispensable
    Backbone of Voluntary Action: Measuring and Valuing the*

Contribution of Older Volunteers, VITA and Volunteering England, London.

21 WRVS and CSV (2006), *Age Shall Not Weary Them Nor the Years Condemn: Retired and Senior Volunteering today,* London.

22 Metropolitan Jewish Health System (2003): *An Evaluation of Elderplan's Time Dollar Model,* New York.

Chapter 3

1   Nick Davies (2005), 'Life on the breadline', *Guardian,* 2 Nov.

2   *Guardian* (2003), 24 Dec.

3   Age Concern England (2007), *Political Bulletin,* May.

4   BBC News (2006), 24 Feb.

5   Help the Aged (2006), *Decent Homes and Fuel Poverty: An Analysis Based on the English House Conditions Survey,* London.

6   Mullan, P. (2002), *The Imaginary Time bomb: Why an Ageing Population Is Not a Social Problem,* London, I B Tauris.

7   Department of Work and Pensions (2002), *Simplicity, Security and Choice: Working and Saving for Retirement.* HMSO, London.

8   Joseph Rowntree Foundation (2004), *From Welfare to Well-being: Planning for an Ageing Society,* Summary conclusions of the Joseph Rowntree Foundation Task Group on Housing, Money and Care for Older People, York.

9   Ibid.

10 *Scotsman* (2004), 11 Oct.

11 BBC News (2007), 'Guide to Europe's pension woes. Who is going to pay for the retirement of future generations?', 17 Aug.

12 Ibid.

13 Ibid.

14 Heller, Peter S. (2003), *Who Will Pay? Coping with Ageing Societies, Climate Change and Other Long-term Fiscal Challenges,* International Monetary Fund, Washington, DC.

15 Joe Harris (2003), *Exploding the Myths: The Truth Behind the State Pension Debate*, London.

16 Will Hutton (2005), 'The British workers' revolution has begun and is changing life for all of us', *Observer*, 4 Dec.

17 Stephen King (2005), 'This debate is about politics, not economics', *Independent*, 28 Nov.

18 Mike Brewer *et al.* (2007), *Pensioner Poverty over the Next Decade: What Role for Tax and Benefit Reform?* Institute for Fiscal Studies, London.

Chapter 4

1 Joseph Rowntree Foundation: *From Welfare to Well-being: Planning for an Ageing Society,* Summary conclusions of the Joseph Rowntree Foundation Task Group on Housing, Money and Care for Older People, York, October 2004

2 Wu, G. Zhao, F. Zhou X,. *et al.* (2002), 'Improvement of isokinetic knee extensor strength and postural sway in the elderly from long term Tai-Chi exercise', *Arch Phys Med Rehabil,* 83(10): pp. 1364–9.

3 Help the Aged (2007), *Taking Control of Incontinence: Exploring the Links with Social Isolation,* London.

4 David Smith (2006), 'Why we're losing our loos', *Observer*, 16 Jul.

5 George Melly (2005), *Slowing Down,* with drawings by Maggi Hambling, Viking, London.

6   David Smith (2006), 'Why we're losing our loos', *Observer,* 16 Jul.

7   Help the Aged (2007), *Nowhere to Go*, London.

8   *Northwich Guardian* (2007), 12 Jun.

9   Anne Karpf (2006), 'I'll fight for a woman's right to pee', *Guardian*, 25 Mar.

10 Rosemary Behan (2007), 'Outrageous: It's no john, no john, no john, no', *The Times*, 11 Jun.

11 Sophie Handler (2006), *The Fluid Pavement and Other Stories on Growing Old in Newham*, London.

12 Ibid.

13 Select Committee on Environment, Transport and Regional Affairs (2001), *Eleventh Report,* May.

14 CABE (2005), *What Are We Scared Of?* London.

15 Nick Butterworth, *Percy the Park Keeper* – various titles, HarperCollins, London.

16 CABE (2005), *Parks Need a Parkforce,* London.

17 English Heritage (2005), *The Park Keeper*, London.

18 Julian Hine and Fiona Mitchell (2001), The Role of Transport in Social Exclusion in Urban Scotland, Development Department Research Programme Research Findings No. 110.

19 Claudia Botham and Tristan Lumley (2004), *Grey Matters: Growing Older in Deprived Areas – a Guide for Donors and Grant-makers,* New Philanthropy Capital, London.

20 Department of Health (2006), *Our Health, Our Care, Our Say: A New Direction for Community Services.* London.

21 BBC News online (2006), 19 May.

22 Royal Town Planning Institute website.

23 Helen Hamlyn Foundation (1986), New Design for Old: an exhibition of new products designed to help older people stay independent at home, Boilerhouse, Victoria and Albert Museum, London.

Chapter 5

1 *The Times* (2007), 1 Nov.
2 Claudia Botham and Tristan Lumley (2004), *Grey Matters: Growing Older in Deprived Areas – a Guide for Donors and Grant-makers,* New Philanthropy Capital, London.
3 Mark Gould (2006), 'Voices of experience', *Guardian,* 1 Feb.
4 National Statistics (2005), *Focus on Older People,* London.
5 Chartered Institute of Library and Information Professionals (2003), *Library and Information Services for Older People: Professional Guidance, Policy and Research,* London.
6 Warwick University (2000), *Making a Difference: Better Government for Older People Evaluation Report.*
7 Rebecca Linley (2000), 'Open to all? The public library and social exclusion', Vol. 3, Working Paper 16, *Public Libraries, Older People and Social Exclusion.*
8 Ibid.
9 Gertrud Seidmann (2006), 'Thunder, lightning and a ray of sunshine: The Rev. Greville John Chester addresses his congregation', *Romulus: Voices,* Wolfson College, Oxford.
10 BBC News (2004), 10 Dec.
11 *Guardian* (2007), 28 Mar.
12 Department for Innovation, Universities and Skills (2007), *World Class Skills: Implementing the Leitch Review of Skills in England,* HMSO, London.
13 Helen Thomas: http://dance.gold.ac.uk/activites.html
14 Voluntary Arts Scotland (2005), *Newsletter,* 15 Jul.
15 *Guardian* (2006), 7 Mar.
16 Giles Hattersley (2007), 'What big downloads you have, grandma', *Sunday Times,* 4 Feb.
17 *Guardian* (2006), 10 Feb.

18 Blake Morrison (2005), *Things My Mother Never Told Me*,
Vintage, London.

19 WRVS (2004), *Society Must Challenge Loneliness and Save
Lives*, London.

20 Ibid.

21 *Guardian* (2006), 12 Apr.

22 *Scotsman* (2006), 1 Jun.

23 *Sydney Morning Herald* (2006), 6 May.

24 Roger Brown (2001), 'Intergenerational Learning in
International Baccalaureate Schools', *IB Research Notes*, Vol. 1,
issue 2, International Baccalaureate Organisation, Bath.

Chapter 6

1   Joseph Rowntree Foundation (2004), *From Welfare to Well-
being: Planning for an Ageing Society,* Summary conclusions
of the Joseph Rowntree Foundation Task Group on Housing,
Money and Care for Older People, York.

2   Department for Business, Enterprise and Regulatory Reform
(2007), *The UK Fuel Poverty Strategy Fifth Annual Progress
Report*, London, HMSO.

3   Joseph Comrie (2004), 'African Caribbean elders and their
housing experiences', *Research Findings*, University of Leeds.

4   Malcolm Harrison (1992), 'Housing association schemes
targeted on black and minority ethnic communities: some
issues of design, security and development', *Social Policy and
Sociology Research Working Paper 5*, University of Leeds.

5   Malcolm Harrison, with Phillips, D., Chahal, K., Hunt, L., and
Perry, J. (2005), 'Revisiting housing need', in *Housing, Race
and Community Cohesion*, Chartered Institute of Housing,
London.

6   Margaret Edwards and Ed Harding (2006), *Building our Futures*: *Meeting the Housing Needs of an Ageing Population*, International Longevity Centre, London.

7   Help the Aged (2006), Sep.

8   Joseph Rowntree Foundation (2006), *Housing with Care for Later Life: A Literature Review*, York, Feb.

9   *The Times* (2006), 24 Oct.

10 *The Times* (2006), 24 Oct.

11 *Lifetime Homes, Lifetime Neighbourhoods: A National Strategy for Housing in an Ageing Society*, DCLG, 2008.

12 Croucher, Pleace and Bevan (2003), *Living at Hartrigg Oaks*, Joseph Rowntree Foundation, York.

13 *Glasgow Herald* (2004), 23 Jun.

14 Neasa MacErlean (2004), 'When is a commune not a commune?', *Observer*, 30 May.

Chapter 7

1   Dee Sedgwick (2006), private letter, 29 May.

2   Janice Robinson and Penny Banks (2005), *The Business of Caring: The Report of the King's Fund Inquiry into Care Services for Older People in London*, King's Fund, London.

3   The Health Service Ombudsman (2003), *NHS Funding for Long Term Care*, HC 399, HMSO, London.

4   Spain coalition (2005), *What Price Care in Old Age?* London. Spain stands for the Social Policy on Ageing Information Network. The charities involved include: Age Concern England, Help the Aged, Alzheimer's Society, Abbeyfield Society, Anchor Trust, Arthritis Care, Association of Charity Officers, Association of Retired Persons Over 50, Beth Johnson Foundation, Carers UK, Centre for Policy on Ageing,

Action on Elder Abuse, Counsel and Care, Fawcett Society,
Greater London Forum for the Elderly, Hanover Housing
Association, Health and Older People, Hill Homes, Jewish
Care, MHA Care Group, National Association of Citizen's
Advice Bureaux, National Pensioners Convention, Parkinsons
Disease Society, RADAR, Relatives and Residents Association,
Senior Citizens Forums Network, The Leveson Centre,
VOICES.

5 Ibid.
6 BBC News (2006), 27 Mar.
7 David Brindle (2007), 'A home care storm brews on the
   horizon', *Guardian*, 3 Jan.
8 Commission for Social Care Inspection (2008), *The State of
   Social Care in England 2006–07*, London.
9 *Scotsman* (2007), 30 Mar.
10 King's Fund (2006), *Wanless Social Care Review: Securing
   Good Care for Older People*, King's Fund, London.
11 Joseph Rowntree Foundation (2006), *The Material Resources
   and Well-being of Older People*, York.
12 *Guardian* (2008), 29 Jan.
13 *Daily Mail* (2007), 30 Jul.
14 *Guardian* (200), 6 Jan.
15 Murray, Jenni (2007), 'My hardest goodbyes', *Daily Mail*, 12 Jul.
16 *Guardian* (2005), 19 Jan.
17 *Scotland on Sunday* (2007), 18 Mar.
18 *Independent* (2006), 19 Aug.
19 *Daily Mail* (2007), 12 Feb.
20 Mary Riddell (2007), 'But not everyone can grow old
   gracefully', *Observer*, 10 Jun.
21 *Observer* (2007), 18 Mar.
22 BBC News (2001), 1 Sep.

23 Melanie Phillips (2003), 'And we call this a welfare state?', *Daily Mail*, 9 Jul.

24 King's Fund (2001), *Future Imperfect?* London.

25 Janet Street-Porter (2004), 'I'll do anything except go into a care home', *Independent*, 6 Feb.

26 *Daily Mail* (2007), 27 Mar.

27 Christopher Manthorp (2006), 'Residential homes aren't always where the heart is', *Guardian*, 8 Feb.

28 Patients Association (2007), *Pain in Older People: A Hidden Problem*, London.

29 Jackie Morris (2007), 'Old age is a marathon', presentation for the JCC and LJCC, 21 Mar.

30 *Guardian* (2007), 2 Apr.

31 *Independent* (2006), 11 Apr.

32 Jay Rayner (2006), 'Hospital food: it's enough to make you sick', *Observer Food Magazine*, Sept.

33 BBC News online (2006), 22 Feb.

34 Fran Abrams (2006), 'Care for the elderly that is very hard to swallow', *The Times*, 3 Jun.

35 European Nutrition for Health Alliance (2005), *Malnutrition Within an Ageing Population*.

36 Ibid.

37 House of Commons (2006), *Hansard Debates*, 8 Feb.

38 *Sunday Telegraph* (2005), 22 May.

39 Marianne Falconer and Desmond O'Neill (2007), 'Out with "the old", elderly and aged', *BMJ*, 10 Feb.

40 English Community Care Association (2006), *Well Watered Residents and Staff?*, 18 Aug.

41 Debbie Andalo (2007), 'Historic changes: charting the past life of care home residents with Alzheimer's can transform occupational therapy', *Guardian*, 17 Jan.

42 English Community Care Association (2006), *What Can We do to Make It Better?*, 28 Mar.

43 Help the Aged (2006), *My Home Life: Quality of Life in Care Homes,* London.

44 Christopher Manthorp (2006), 'Size really does matter on the home front', *Society Guardian*, 8 Nov.

45 BBC News (2006), 11 Nov.

46 Help the Aged 'Help Stop Elder Abuse' website.

47 Alexander Chancellor (2007), 'The elderly are being robbed and exploited. And it's their grasping children who are targeting them', *Guardian*, 23 Feb.

48 Commission for Social Care Inspection (2008), *The State of Social Care in England 2006–07,* London.

Chapter 8

1   Muriel Gillick (2006), *The Denial of Ageing: Perpetual Youth, Eternal Life, and Other Dangerous Fantasies*, Harvard University Press, Cambridge, Massachusetts, and London.

2   Gomes, B., and Higginson, I. (2006), 'Factors influencing death at home in terminally ill patients with cancer systematic review,' *British Medical Journal*, 8 Feb.

3   Muriel Gillick (2006), *The Denial of Ageing: Perpetual Youth, Eternal Life, and Other Dangerous Fantasies*, Harvard University Press, Cambridge, Massachusetts, and London.

4   *Sunday Telegraph* (2008), 27 Jan; and *Daily Mail* (2008), 28 Jan.

5   Help the Aged (2007), *Too Old: Older People's Accounts of Discrimination, Exclusion and Rejection*, London.

6   Ibid.

7   Ibid.

8 Rudd, A.G., Hoffman, A., Down, C., Pearson, M. and Lowe, D. (2007), 'Access to stroke care in England, Wales and Northern Ireland: the effects of age, gender and weekend admission', *Age and Ageing*, 14 Mar.

9 Help the Aged (2007), *Too Old: Older People's Accounts of Discrimination, Exclusion and Rejection*, London.

10 Harries, C., Forrest, D., Harvey, N., McLelland, A., and Bowling, A. (2007), 'Which doctors are influenced by a patient's age? A multi-method study of angina treatment in general practice, cardiology and gerontology', *Quality and Safer Health Care*, 1623–7.

11 Sampson E.L., Gould, V., Lee, D., and Blanchard, B. (2006), 'Differences in care received by patients with and without dementia who died during acute hospital admission: a retrospective case study', *Age and Ageing*, 35: 187–9.

12 Help the Aged (2007), *Spotlight Report 2007: Spotlight on Older People in the UK*, London.

13 *Daily Mail* (2007), 12 Jun.

14 CSCI (2006), *Supporting People, Promoting Independence*, London.

15 *Guardian* (2006), 2 May.

16 National Primary Care Research and Development Centre (2006), *Evaluation of the Evercare Approach to Case Management of Frail Elderly People*, Manchester.

17 Morris, J., Beaumont, D., and Oliver, D. (2006), 'Decent health care for older people', *BMJ*, 332: 1166–8, 20 May.

18 Ian Philp (2006), *A New Ambition for Old Age: Next Steps in Implementing the National Service Framework*, Department of Health, London.

19 Morris, J., Beaumont, D., and Oliver, D. (2006), 'Decent health care for older people', *BMJ*, 332: 1166–8, 20 May.

20 Ibid.

21 Ian Philp (2006), *A New Ambition for Old Age: Next Steps in Implementing the National Service Framework*, Department of Health, London.

22 Morris, J., Beaumont, D., and Oliver, D. (2006), 'Decent health care for older people', *BMJ*, 332: 1166–8, 20 May.

23 Ian Philp (2006), *A New Ambition for Old Age: Next Steps in Implementing the National Service Framework*, Department of Health, London.

24 Yvonne Roberts (2006), 'Why my father deserves to have his lost voice back', *Observer*, 22 Jan.

25 National Audit Office (2007), *Improving Services for People with Dementia*, 4 Jul, HC 604 Session 2006–7.

26 National Institute for Clinical Excellence (2006), *Dementia: Supporting People with Dementia and Their Carers in Health and Social Care*, NICE Clinical Guideline 42.

27 National Audit Office (2007), *Improving Services for People with Dementia*, 4 Jul, HC 604 Session 2006–7.

28 National Institute for Clinical Excellence (2006), *Dementia: Supporting People with Dementia and Their Carers in Health and Social Care*, NICE Clinical Guideline 42.

29 Ros Levenson (1998), *Drugs and Dementia: A Guide to Good Practice in the Use of Neuroleptic Drugs in Care Homes for Older People*, Age Concern, London.

30 *Guardian* (2007), 30 Mar.

31 Ibid.

32 Age Concern and Mental Health Foundation (2003), *UK Inquiry into Mental Health and Well-being in Later Life*, London.

33 Department of Health (2007), news release, 3 and 6 Aug; Gateway reference: 8634.

34 National Audit Office (2007), *Improving Services for People with Dementia*, 4 Jul, HC 604 Session 2006–7.

35 Age Concern and Mental Health Foundation (2003), *UK Inquiry into Mental Health and Well-being in Later Life*, London.

36 MIND (2005), *Access All Ages Campaign: Mental Health Needs in Later Life Must Be Met, Not Marginalised*, London.

37 *Daily Mail* (2007), 14 Aug.

38 Age Concern and Mental Health Foundation (2003), *UK Inquiry into Mental Health and Well-being in Later Life*, London.

39 Mary Godfrey with Tracy Denby (2004), *Depression and Older People: Towards Securing Well-being in Later Life*, Help the Aged, London.

40 Derek Beeston (2007), 'Sad ending', *Guardian*, 14 Mar.

41 Hazel Heath (2006), *Specialist Community Nurses for Older People at Home: A Report on the Feasibility of the Role*, Clore Duffield Foundation, London.

42 Ros Levenson (2006), 'Lessons from the end of a life', *BMJ*, 20 Mar.

43 BBC News (2005), 20 Jul.

44 Ibid.

45 http://hellsgeriatrics.co.uk/gret-matters-abuse.htm

46 *Mirror* (2006), 23 Feb.

47 Jo Revill (2007), 'The dirty truth on the wards', *Observer*, 14 Oct.

48 Ibid.

49 BBC News online (2006), 28 Aug.

50 Age Concern (2006), *Hungry to Be Heard: The Scandal of Malnourished Older People in Hospital*, London.

51 Ian Philp (2006), *A New Ambition for Old Age: Next Steps in Implementing the National Service Framework*, Department of Health, London.

52 AlisonTonks (1999), 'Medicine must change to serve an ageing society: eradicate age discrimination and increase resources', *BMJ*, 319: 1450–51, 4 Dec.

Chapter 9

1 This introduction was adapted from my article in *Health Service Journal*, 3 Oct 1996.

2 Melanie Phillips (2004), 'Love and dignity inextricably mixed', *Jewish Chronicle*, 13 Aug.

3 Rosemary Dinnage (1992), *The Ruffian on the Stair*, Penguin, London.

4 Diana Athill (2007), *Somewhere Near the End,* Granta Books, London.

5 *Guardian,* 22 February 2006

6 Diana Athill (2007), *Somewhere Near the End,* Granta Books, London.

7 Kate Berridge (2001), *Vigor Mortis: The End of the Death Taboo*, Profile, London.

8 Tom Owen (ed.) (2005), *Dying in Older Age: Reflections and Experiences from an Older Person's Perspective*, Help the Aged, London.

9 Iona Joy and Sarah Sandford (2004), *Caring about Dying: Palliative Care and Support for the Terminally Ill – a Guide for Donors and Grant-makers*, New Philanthropy Capital, London.

10 *British Medical Journal* (2003), 'What is a good death?', no. 7408, 26 Jul.

11 Peter Jupp and Clare Gittings (1999), *Death in England: An Illustrated History*, Manchester University Press, Manchester.

12 Samuel Belgradi (1976), *Hebrew Ethical Wills*, edited by Israel Abrahams, Jewish Publication Society of America, Philadelphia, pp. 259ff.

13 Gomes, B. and Higginson, I. (2006), 'Factors influencing death at home in terminally ill patients with cancer systematic review', *British Medical Journal*, 8 Feb.

14 Jonathan Wittenberg (2006), 'The last word', *Jewish Chronicle*, 13 Jan.

15 Muriel Gillick (2006), *The Denial of Ageing: Perpetual Youth, Eternal Life, and Other Dangerous Fantasies*, Harvard University Press Cambridge, Massachusetts, and London.

16 Age Concern (1999), *Debate of the Age*, Health and Care Study Group, London.

Chapter 10

1 *The Times* (2006), 24 Aug.

2 *Metro* (2007), 6 Feb.

3 *Camden New Journal* (2008), 7 Feb.

4 *The Times* (2006), 21 Dec.

5 *Irish Times* (2007), 12 Sep.

6 *Community Care* (2007), 6 Sep.

7 BBC News (2004), 29 Nov.

8 Kate Zernike (2007), 'The body may age, but romance stays fresh', *New York Times*, 25 Nov.

9 *The Times* (2007), 23 Aug.

10 Virginia Ironside (2006), 'How to grow old disgracefully', *Independent*, 19 Sep.

11 Ibid.

12 Joan Bakewell (2006), *The View from Here: Life at Seventy*, Atlantic Books, London.

13 Ibid.

14 Shirley Toulson (1998), *The Country of Old Age: A Personal Adventure in Time*, Hodder & Stoughton, London.

15 Charles Williams (1937), *Descent into Hell*, London.

16 Andrew Powell (2006), 'Spirituality and later life', *Bishop John Robinson Newsletter*, no. 17, May.

17 Mary Riddell (2007), 'But not everyone can grow old gracefully', *Observer*, 10 Jun.

18 Richard Hoggart (2005), *Promises to Keep: Thoughts in Old Age*, Continuum, London.

19 Michael Kimmelman (2006), 'Goya, unflinching, defied old age', *New York Times*, 24 Feb.

20 BBC News (2004), 12 Jul.

21 Sinclair, David, Swan, Amy, and Pearson, Anna (2007), *Social Inclusion and Older People: A Call for Action*, Help the Aged, London.

22 BBC News (2007), 19 Jul.

23 *Daily Telegraph* (2006), 27 Jun.

24 BBC News (2007), 14 Jan.

25 Raymond Tallis (2006), 'To the barricades, old codgers: you're the last bastions of threatened liberty', *The Times*, 31 Jul.

Bibliography

Asato, Jessica: *Fit for the Future – A New Vision for Older People's Care and Support*, Counsel and Care, 2006

Athill, Diana: *Somewhere Towards the End*, Granta Books, London, 2008

Bakewell, Joan: *The View from Here – Life at Seventy*, Atlantic Books, London, 2006

Berridge, Kate: *Vigor Mortis – the End of the Death Taboo*, Profile, London, 2001

Blaikie, Andrew: *Ageing and Popular Culture*, Cambridge University Press, 1999

Butterworth, Nick: *Percy the Park Keeper* – various titles, HarperCollinsChildrensBooks, London.

Carter, Sydney: Run the Film Backwards, a poem, from Sydney Carter's *Lord of the Dance and Other Songs and Poems*, Stainer and Bell, London, 2002

Clarke, Alison: *Showing Restraint*, Counsel and Care, London, 2002

Department of Health: *Care Homes for Older People – National Minimum Standards*, Stationery Office, London, 2003

Dinnage, Rosemary: *The Ruffian on the Stair*, Penguin, London, 1990

Fearnley-Whittingstall, Jane: *The Good Granny Guide, or How to Be a Modern Grandmother*, Short Books, London, 2005

Gillick, Muriel R.: *Choosing Medical Care in Old Age – What Kind? How Much? When to Stop?*, Harvard University Press, Cambridge, Mass. and London, 1994

————— : *The Denial of Aging: Perpetual Youth, Eternal Life, and Other Dangerous Fantasies*, Harvard University Press, Cambridge, Mass. and London, 2006

The Health Service Ombudsman, *NHS Funding for Long Term Care*, HC 399, Stationery Office Books, 2003

Hoggart, Richard: *Promises to Keep: Thoughts in Old Age*, Continuum, London, 2005

Huber, J. and Skidmore, P.: *The New Old – Why Baby Boomers Won't Be Pensioned Off*, Demos, London, 2003

Hyams, Jacky: *Time to Help Your Parents – A Practical Guide to Recognising Problems and Providing Support*, Piatkus Books, London, 2007

Ironside, Virginia: *No, I Don't Want to Join a Book Club – Diary of a Sixtieth Year*, Penguin, London, 2007

Johnston, Susanna (ed.): *Late Youth: An Anthology Celebrating the Joys of Being Over Fifty*, Arcadia, London, 2005

Joy, Iona and Sandford, Sarah: *Caring about Dying: Palliative Care and Support for the Terminally Ill – A Guide for Donors and Grant-makers*: New Philanthropy Capital, London, 2004

Joy, Iona and Fradd, Adrian: *Striking a Chord – Who is Using Music*, New Philanthropy Capital, London, 2006

Jupp, Peter C. and Gittings, Clare: *Death in England – An Illustrated History*, Manchester University Press, Manchester, 1999

Lacheze, Marie: *Choices for Later Life: Making the Most of Life After 50*, Piatkus, London, 2007

Marcus, Nella J: *Fifty Plus*, Macdonald Optima, London, 1991

Melly, George: *Slowing Down*, Viking, London, 2005

Morrison, Blake: *Things My Mother Never Told Me*, Vintage,
    London, 2005
Mullan, Phil: *The Imaginary Time Bomb – Why an Ageing
    Population is Not a Social Problem*, I B Tauris, London, 1999
Neuberger, Julia: *The Moral State We're In*, HarperCollins,
    London, 2005
Roth, Philip: *Everyman*, Jonathan Cape, London, 2006
Rowe, J. W. and Kahn, R. L.: *Successful Aging*, Pantheon Books,
    New York, 1998
Sackville-West, Vita: *All Passion Spent*, Virago, London, 1985
Shea, Michael: *The Freedom Years – Tactical Tips for the
    Trailblazer Generation*, Capstone, Chichester, 2006
Shoard, Marion: *A Survival Guide to Later Life (Daily Telegraph)*,
    Robinson Publishing, London, 2004
Thane, Pat: *Old Age in English History*, Oxford University Press,
    Oxford, 2000
—— (ed): *The Long History of Old Age*, Thames and Hudson,
    London, 2005
Toulson, Shirley: *The Country of Old Age – A Personal Adventure
    in Time*, Hodder and Stoughton, London, 1998
Whitehorn, Katharine: *Selective Memory – An Autobiography*,
    Virago, London, 2007

Index